The **DOCTOR** of **ADDICTIONS**

*Dr. Kishore's Breakthrough in Addiction
Treatment, and the Tragic Story of
How the Deep State Destroyed It*

JOEL MCDURMON

DEVOTED BOOKS

DALLAS, GEORGIA

The Doctor of Addictions
*Dr. Kishore's Breakthrough in Addiction Treatment, and
the Tragic Story of How the Deep State Destroyed It*

Published by:
>   *Devoted Books*
>   P.O. Box 371
>   Braselton, GA 30517

Printed in the United States of America.

ISBN: 9781674461519

To

Kishore

for never giving up

Other books
by Joel McDurmon:

The Problem of Slavery in Christian America

The Bible & War in America

Restoring America One County at a Time

*The Bounds of Love: An Introduction to
God's Law of Liberty*

Available at www.Amazon.com

CONTENTS

Foreword

by Rev. Dr. Samuel B. Hogan

Dr. Joel McDurmon is a gifted theologian who presents truth in a dramatically interpretive way. He has written a provocative, semibiographical story of a man seeking to change the treatment of addiction.

He portrays Dr. Kishore's birth, life, and professional career and how they played a part in developing his revolutionary approach to substance use disorders.

Kishore's treatment process brings hope for a change, not just another alternative drug that continues the vicious cycle.

One would assume there would be universal excitement to see new methods of treatment, giving genuine hope to our suffering brothers and sisters.

However, each chapter will bring you closer to the understanding of how a man of his knowledge, gifts, and calling can be shut down and publicly destroyed by many of the powers that be—even when addiction is one of the significant ills affecting our society today.

Many advocates' attempts genuinely to help those with substance use disorders fail when they are drawn by the irresistible attraction of money derived from mainstream methods of revolving door treatments.

Dr. McDurmon's book exposes the breakthrough treatment methods and the tenacious battle of Dr. Kishore against the vested interests.

REV. DR. SAMUEL B. HOGAN, SR.
Bishop of the First Jurisdiction of Massachusetts,
Church of God in Christ, Inc.
Counselor and Instructor, Harvard Divinity School

Preface

"**I** would have been dead," the voice told me confidently across the phone. Virtually every testimony from former patients contains that line. "If it weren't for him, I would have been dead."

In this case, the voice belonged to Jay Lafauci, a former fire lieutenant in Melrose, Massachusetts, a middle-class community north of Boston. Like millions of victims of the opioid epidemic, Jay's trouble resulted after a personal injury. He hurt his back. A doctor prescribed him opioid painkillers—Percocet® and Oxycontin®. Like so many others in the 1990s, his doctor overprescribed these addictive drugs. "You got cancer?" his pharmacist quipped, goggling the size of the order. But it was just back pain. Like many others, Jay would get hooked. When his prescriptions ran out, he could not quit. In what is a tragically common story now, Jay found what he wanted on the street.

He knew he needed to quit. Over the following years, like most others, Jay checked into rehab "like 20 times," he said. But detox is only a seven-day stint—not long enough, not comprehensive enough for sobriety. "Spin dry," Jay called it. Once out, patients cannot hold out long. Most inevitably return to substance abuse.

Inevitably, Jay got busted. "If you do something illegal long enough," he confessed, allowing me to fill in the blank. He had to resign his job with the fire department. He was broke. He lost nearly everything. Eventually, detox itself was no longer an option. Insurance companies will quit paying it. But there was still one other option. Insurance said it would still pay for primary care, and there was an outlier in the Boston area treating addiction as outpatient primary care. Jay's insurance company told him to go to this guy.

"But it's a Saturday night?" Jay thought, "What doctor is open at these hours?" He called anyway. It turned out, that doctor took calls and in fact took patients almost any time. His name is Punyamurtula Kishore (rhymes with "sea-shore"), and he is known to many of his patients and friends as "The Doctor of Addictions."

Thanks to Dr. Kishore's pioneering genius and tireless efforts, Jay achieved a lasting sobriety. Today, he has been sober for 16 years, and works as a bus driver. "If it were not for him," Jay said, "I would have been dead. I am thankful to this day."[1]

You can hear the confession, "I would have been dead were it not for him," repeated on the lips of many of Kishore's former patients. One posted in a forum with the same story of having failed after detox multiple times, never lasting longer than 12 days. After Kishore's treatments, however, he was transformed. He wanted to share his story with the world: "As far as I'm concerned, this man is a genius! . . . I owe my life to him!"[2]

Kerri Hume, the office manager of Kishore's Weymouth clinic stated, "So many were getting their lives back on track, getting good jobs, able to go back to their families."[3] Staff nurse Luz Thomas recalled one occasion when a former patient's wife brought a cake into the clinic to celebrate two years of sobriety. Luz said, "This man had been on Methadone for 20 years of his life and he was free, completely free from everything, and he was living just such a

---

1. All of Jay Lafauci's statements are from a private interview by the author, December 4, 2019.

2. Shared with the author via private email.

3. This and several of the following testimonies were compiled by Joaquin Fernandez, co-producer of a forthcoming documentary about Kishore, *Hero In America*.

marvelous life and they were celebrating." Another former patient named Gena said, "When I was 19, I couldn't get sober for more than . . . I think three weeks was the longest I had gone in years. . . . I honestly don't think I'd be alive to see my son right now. . . ."

Union presence is powerful in Massachusetts, and unions rely on workers. But the middle-class, blue-collar workforce was being decimated by the opioid epidemic. One top official, however, learned of Kishore's success, and he became a top fan. Former state senator Steven Tolman is president of the Massachusetts AFL-CIO. He speaks highly of the Doctor of Addictions: "When I had the cases where nothing was working, I would call Dr. Kishore, and he would say, send them right over. I'll see him. . . . He would never say no. He would always see the patient and he would talk to the patient in his gentle manner and he would explain to them that 'you can beat this. You don't have to be on dangerous drugs. You can get off this. You might be sick for a while, but you can beat this.'"

With the opioid crisis spiraling into a well-publicized epidemic, you would think Kishore's name and his unique, powerful methods would be a household name—like "AA" or the standard mass-produced answer of methadone clinics. During his most active years, he treated hundreds of thousands of addicted patients in Massachusetts and achieved sobriety rates unheard-of among the now-traditional narcotic models, which Kishore refers to as "legal dope." The model he developed after decades of research, education, and practice, rises as a beacon of hope amidst our epidemic today. It is time to look beyond the obviously failed detox and meth-clinic paradigms and pay attention to a *proven* better way.

***

When I finally met Dr. Kishore in person, I was unprepared for one of the gentlest, kindest, and most humble men ever to enter my 45 years of experience. I had spoken with him on the phone, corresponded with him, read about his practice and his case, and written articles about him. I knew he was professional, rigorous, scientific, and in command of the rare and difficult medical specialty of addiction treatment. When we met in person, I anticipated something of a commanding expert shaped by decades of working with addictions, drug dealers, prisoners, business regulators, medical boards, insurance companies, lawyers, politicians, and other cutthroats—the kind of experience that can leave one not only seasoned but hardened, even cynical. Yet across from me sat a warm, gentle man with soft eyes, graceful manners, and a consistent, calm, humble voice. I kept reminding myself that this man almost singlehandedly pioneered a revolution in a medical field. His advances in addiction treatment produced sobriety rates unseen anywhere else before or since.

For about thirty minutes, Kishore engaged me with descriptions of medical details that would probably have been boring had anyone else related them; but a love for his practice, like the devotion of a missionary, exuded through his ever-calm voice with such passion that I could not stop listening.

The relationship that developed that day led to an admiration. The more I studied the man, his life, his practice, and his story, the more I realized what a rare opportunity this was in so many ways. Not many men of this character and caliber come along. You are about to read about a man who survived from his very birth through a miracle, grew into a star pupil in India, became a doctor, came to the U.S., landed by the hand of providence in an addiction care hospital, studied further at Harvard University, worked with world-renowned physicians and professors, became a medical director of multiple hospitals and medical programs, directed the medical care of a whole state's correctional institutions, opened his own private practice, revolutionized addiction treatment, attained unheard-of sobriety rates, grew his business from a single office into 52 clinics with 370 employees and $20 million in revenue, donated 30 percent of his own salary to an educational charity he created, treated over a quarter of a million addicted individuals and their families, was honored with awards from all kinds of hospitals, professional groups, professional sports teams, and much more, and . . .

. . . there he sat speaking to me as if I were his peer, on his level, a casual friend.

I can honestly say I have rarely if ever met such genius, grit, gentleness, accomplishment, and humility in a single individual.

Kishore's rise from humble beginnings in India to some of the most prestigious medical establishments in Boston (or the world, for that matter) constitutes a realization of the American dream extended to an international level. It is an idyllic path, not only as a personal success, but even more so when we consider the long record of personalized and effective care focused on patients. It is the American dream *and* the moral ideal of putting others first, of actually serving people, rolled into one. As one of those things that helps "restore faith in humanity," you cannot ask for much more.

It comes in shocking contrast, then, to picture this same Dr. Kishore at 10:45 p.m. one Tuesday night, jolted by an all-out SWAT raid bursting through his door. One simply cannot imagine armies of black vehicles lining and barricading his street, police surrounding his house, a circling helicopter loudly clapping overhead, and a full act of rudeness inside as Mrs. Kishore was ordered around while the doctor was jostled, handcuffed, stuffed away, and hustled off to jail.

But this is exactly what happened to this man—the man who has done more for the addiction epidemic in America than any other single individual, and would do more still if he could.

What could warrant this treatment? Sure, SWAT raids are indeed overused these days—multiple times per day, and sometimes for things as routine as basic search warrants. But even these are a minority. Was the doctor leading a human trafficking operation? Did he deal in child pornography? Were there ties to organized crime? Did he have a trail of bodies? Was he running illegal narcotics through his operations?

Nothing like these were the case. Nothing. The crime for which Dr. Kishore was later charged? Allegedly running a "kickback scheme"—a charge that was not only was never substantiated, but was easily disproven. Nevertheless, the state would use the charge, and a long line of dirty tricks, to destroy Kishore's practice.

But why? Others had actually settled such charges with mere fines and gone back to work. Someone for some reason wanted something more from Kishore. They wanted him gone—gone as a rival, gone as a thorn in their side, gone as a threat to something they coveted. Or so it seems.

What was it? Something did not add up, and perhaps that is the best phrase to use: numbers not adding up. Numbers, that is, as in cash flow. Kishore's radical success in actually sobering-up addicted patients, and *without* addictive medications, meant several powerful forces were losing out on streams of potential revenue.

This brief biography lays out just a bit of that story and some of the understanding behind it. We will get a glimpse how so many powerful forces get filthy rich from the addiction industry, why such an industry has a powerful interest in keeping millions of people addicted to "treatment" prescription drugs, and why actually doing something to solve the opioid epidemic, as well as other addictions, is actually perceived as a threat by some entities.

It is my hope that my meager contribution may have several beneficial effects. First, it will complement the work of others on Kishore's case. There is a set of more detailed articles prepared by the Chalcedon Foundation, and a documentary coming soon on the same subject: the reader can see my recommended resources in the back. Second, I hope that those affected by addiction will learn there is a better way than trading one addiction for another, and that the aspiration of *many* addicted individuals for actual sobriety can indeed be a reality, and very effectively so through the methods Kishore pioneered and refined over decades. Third, I hope to augment the growing realization that while health industry lobbies and centralized government are each proper enough objects of criticism as they are, they make for an even more toxic combination. The results have been an increase in addictions, debt, prisoners, and probationers while the epidemic still spirals out of control. Finally, I hope that highlighting these realities will inspire some policymakers and politicians to speak the truth and do the right thing—which will very likely be an act of political self-immolation. Nevertheless, our country and her 20 million addicted individuals plea for voices that will brave the flames.

I have to add a note about the use of the terms "addict," "addicted persons," or the like. Some leaders in the substance abuse treatment community have begun a campaign to shift away from the word "addict." These propose using "people-first" language which does not seem to define people by their disorder, focuses on the medical nature of the condition, and seeks to use only language which promotes recovery. While these are certainly notable ideals with which I and the subject of this book agree, it is nevertheless sometimes difficult to tell where they truly benefit the patients as opposed to where they merely serve certain aims of political correctness or even parts of the industry itself. I have chosen to retain "addict" and related terms in some places due to the actual meaning of the word: *to yield, surrender, or become enslaved* to something. In one tale, it referred to an ancient Roman slave who had been freed, but who had become so habitualized to his chains that he remained in them anyway. Far from defining the individual by his condition, the term, when it is allowed this fundamental meaning, highlights both the voluntary and involuntary forces at work in substance addiction. Part of the treatment developed by Kishore, as we shall see, requires addressing the condition in these terms.

This book is in no way intended to be a thorough exposé of Kishore's case. It serves only as an introduction to the man himself, his powerful solution to addiction, and the even more powerful forces that took him down. In order to tell that story through the lens of Kishore's life, we will back up and start at the beginning.

JOEL MCDURMON
March, 2020
Dallas, GA

One

Miracle Child

Punyamurtula Subbarao Kishore was born on June 3, 1950, in Kakinada, a deep-water port city of around 100,000 population (nearing 500,000 today) in the state of Andhra Pradesh, India. The Godavari River streamed out just south of town. To the east lay the Bay of Bengal.

For baby Kishore, prospects were both bright and as dark as could be. On the bright side, the child came from a relatively advantageous background. Both of his parents were physicians. His father came from the Brahmin caste, the highest in India, which supplies Hindu priests. Besides priests, a subcaste of Brahmins known as Niyogis became merchants, agriculturalists, or skilled tradesmen, always with the benefit of working from within the highest social class. During the Maratha Imperial rule of the 18th century, many Brahmins were made administrators and bureaucrats. When the British took over the following century, these were adapted quickly to leading positions. They were among the first in India to incorporate western education. For Kishore's father, this translated as a traditional Indian medical education and social status bolstered by the overlay that British rule gave to both.

Even more promise arose from the mother's side. Her father and mother actively embraced the Indian Independence movement under Gandhi. Grandpa Subbarao, from whom baby Kishore would derive his middle name, took part in the widespread illegal salt harvests as a tax revolt against British rule. Indians traditionally collected salt from evaporated sea water. Since the entry of the East India Trading Company in 1835, however, the British ran a monopoly trade on salt and imposed high taxes. During the Spring of 1930, Gandhi engaged in a 240-mile "Salt March" protesting the tax and British rule, and asked all Indian citizens to engage in the act of non-violent civil disobedience. It was a widespread act symbolic in much the same way and for the same reasons as our own Boston Tea Party in America. Grandpa Subbarao was a local exponent of this resistance, and he paid for it, serving time in jail. It was only after Indian independence was long established that his heroism received recognition. At the 25th national anniversary in 1972, the Indian government brought him to Dehli, awarded him the *Tamra Patra* ("Copper Plate") given to Freedom Fighters, and gave him a lifetime pension.

Subbarao not only resisted the British, he would defy some traditional Indian conventions as well. His wife had suffered from health concerns from a very early age. With no education even in literacy, she almost certainly would have faced a traditional arranged marriage designed to get a less favorable prospective wife married off as easily as possible. Subbarao loved her and spared her from such ignominy by doing what was nearly unthinkable at the time: eloping.

He had not only overcome a damaging tradition, he won quite a prize. Despite her apparent ill health, she went on to bear five daughters. In keeping with their enlightened and independent behavior to date, the couple encouraged education even for the girls. The oldest of these, Goteti Seshagiri, would later marry and become Kishore's mother. Some members of the Indian Congress sought to help the Goteti family in part because of Subbarao's faithful resistance to the British, and due to the large amount of farmland he had lost under British persecution and imprisonment. As a result, the children were afforded the opportunity for an education.

Seshasgiri had been inspired by the example of Dr. Dwarkanath Kotnis. He had answered a national call in 1938 to join a medical mission from India to help the Chinese during the second Sino-Japanese War. He dedicated his life to the cause and became a symbol of international humanitarianism and medicine. To this day he is revered still in China and has hospitals named after him. Seshagiri was part of this phenomenon. She was allowed into medical school at age 14, graduated, and was practicing by the time she was 19. She was one of the first six women to become physicians in southeastern India.

Seshagiri's marriage was unorthodox as well. Kishore's father attended medical school, too, but only after a bout with tuberculosis left him in a sanitorium for three years. His schooling was behind, and he fell into the same class as the younger Miss Goteti. The couple lived out a classic romance: boy meets girl, girl asks for help with science experiment; boy answers; boy falls in love with girl. The two decided to get married, again, bucking the tradition of arranged marriages.

The couple graduated and both went into practice. Seshagiri was soon traveling throughout town and countryside delivering babies, performing minor surgeries, and caring for people in a wide radius about Kakinada. She and her husband would later go on to found a hospital in Kakinada, named after Dr. Kotnis. It would operate from around 1950 until 1994.

Kishore, then, would indeed arrive in a world of many advantages, but his story has a less promising side as well. Baby Kishore arrived in this world prematurely by a startling three months. That he survived at all is a miracle. Neonatal intensive care was only beginning to appear in the most advanced hospitals in the West. It would take decades before technology and standards of care developed, and even longer before they were commonplace. In 1950, it was unheard-of in India. Today, a child born at six months, or 24 weeks, is among the earliest that may survive, even with our advanced care. It would have been unthinkable in 1950. The outlook was so bleak that Kishore's mother returned to her medical practice as soon as she was able, leaving the frail start of a child at home with her mother, assuming he would certainly not survive.

Grandmother Goteti may have lacked the ability to read, but she spoke fluently the language of love. She did not give up on tiny Kishore. She nurtured and cared for him with utmost patience and attention. The effort would result in a miracle. Despite the absence of medical technology, the child survived. Eventually he grew as strong as a normal healthy child, and went on to thrive.

His mother likely felt guilty for prematurely abandoning the child, so, from then on, she took him with her everywhere she went. This arrangement quickly provided the young child with an informal medical education. Seshagiri's rounds led him along through huts and small houses in rural villages. They would sometimes drive long distances. By the time he was ten years old, he was aiding her in simple tasks even during surgery. She would have him put on a mask and hold an anesthesia bottle for her. Not only did he gain such unique and valuable experiences, he was also inspired by his mother's passionate and relentless care for others, against social and class norms as well as adverse conditions. "She was very courageous," Kishore recalled.

He also recalled how something in her had changed since he had been born. Kishore recalled both of his parents originally being atheists, but when he was around four years old, she made the decision to enroll him in a private school operated by the Order of the Sisters of St. Joseph. This was very peculiar, he says, because there were other options. Why she chose a Christian school was not clear. It is possible that his near-miraculous survival had stirred something in her.

The effect of the school would be even greater than the mystery of why she chose it. Kishore says, "It made me who I am today." The Sisters taught him English, Bible, art, and all branches of education. He recalls with fondness learning to copy and to write poetry and making pictures. After an initial period of learning to fit in socially, young Kishore launched into a career of academic success and never looked back.

"I won all the awards," Kishore said, as he explained how he had always been the "top student" in school. He did not exaggerate, and the success would only continue. After seven years with the Sisters, he was transferred to public school. He remained a top student. By the time he readied for college, he had won two scholarships in Andhra Pradesh.

Kishore decided to follow the family tradition of medicine, and to this end, took the entry test for medical college. This merit test in India is used to screen those best suited. Students who score highly enough are ranked and awarded corresponding seats in the college. Out of thousands of students vying for seats, Kishore scored 17th in the nation, and was awarded the first seat in his home state at the Andhra Medical College in 1967.

While in school, Kishore not only succeeded, but began to look to his future. He traveled to take an exam offered internationally by the U.S. government. Following the advent of Medicare in 1965, administrators feared a shortage of doctors and moved to attract as many as possible on into the 1970s. One result was an international outreach to discover talented, qualified physicians. Passage of the exam would be rewarded with a lifetime visa. Kishore passed and accepted the prize, but remained unsure of what he wanted to do.

Upon graduating medical school, he fancied the idea of hospital administration. His parents had opened the hospital, so it seemed logical, and he enjoyed it. He could not get away from the formative experience of family practice which he had gained alongside his mother those early years. It was "imprinted on me," he says. His brother, however, was already a practicing surgeon in New Delhi, and he called the new graduate to come enter his training program. Kishore heeded that call.

After a couple years in the surgical program, Kishore decided it was not for him. His brother excelled at surgery, but he did not feel he had the hands for it, and he preferred family practice. Around that same time in 1977, the U.S. government brought an ultimatum. Apparently, many foreign doctors who had passed the exam and received visas nevertheless tarried and never acted upon them. The message came: use it or lose it. Kishore's brother had a contact in Boston who was also a distant relative of the family. Kishore made arrangements and set off. He arrived in the U.S. on the last day before the deadline to keep his visa. He had no idea of the even greater and more improbable events the hand of Providence had prepared ahead of him.

Two

Meetings with Providence

Kishore had made preparations with his Boston contact, Dr. Sonty, to pick him up at the airport, and to provide him a place to stay until he got established. On the day of his arrival, however, Sonty was a no-show. It was then that a random good Samaritan man and woman noticed the Indian stranger tarrying awkwardly. They offered to help him get to his destination.

They took him to Sonty's residence and helped him unload. He went inside briefly and then returned to thank them for their act of kindness, but unfortunately found only his bags unloaded for him and the couple already vanished.

The young man felt like he should try to say thank you, but he had not even gotten their names. He had no address or contact. So, he sat down and wrote a letter to a local paper. The editor of *The Boston Globe* was impressed enough that the letter appeared on page A6, on January 16, 1977:

Helping Hand

I am a physician from India. I arrived here in Boston late on a Saturday night. As a stranger at the airport, I was quite lost. Being in the United States for the first

7

time, I was having a problem in dialing my friend's
number and in seeking transportation to his place.

An old lady and a young man were watching my tra-
vails. Without a request from my side, he volunteered
to take me along in his car and drop me at my relation's
place.

In big cities, we are told, people are impersonal and
aloof. But this nice gesture from those good Bostonians, who names and addresses I do not know, proves
otherwise.

DR. P. S. KISHORE
Boston

This good deed was not only rewarded, but the thanks it received was a good deed that would itself be rewarded by yet another providential event.

The Monday following publication of the letter, Kishore asked
his host how best to go about finding a job in the medical field.
Sonty supplied his young friend with one of those pre-smart-
phone relics known as the Greater Boston Yellow Pages, a heavy
printed directory of phone numbers to area businesses. "Start calling," came the instruction.

Kishore spent the day calling through the alphabetical list of
hospitals in the area. He heard rejection after rejection, until he
got to the very last name at the long list: The Washingtonian Center for Addictions. He was not an addiction specialist yet, but a
family practitioner, but this was his last option.

Surprisingly, the Washingtonian had an opening, but it was not
much. A doctor had taken vacation and the Center needed someone to cover for two weeks. But would Dr. Kishore be a fit? Were
there not many others who could fill a temporary spot more fit-
tingly than an outsider with no specialization in addictions?

The director of the Washingtonian at the time was Dr. David C.
Lewis, who would go on later to hold two professorates at Brown

University, one in Medicine and Community Health and another in Alcohol and Addiction Studies. During the time he was entertaining candidates to fill the meager cover position, he picked up the morning newspaper for a few minutes.

Dr. Kishore's fortune had fallen out rapidly along a timeline of events over a mere ten or so days, and in a way no human could have planned or expected. He had landed in Boston on January 8. He wrote his thank you note about the anonymous couple to the paper the next day. On Wednesday, January 12, the paper called him to verify the story, and said they would publish it. It appeared in the paper the following Sunday. It was that very paper which Dr. Lewis picked up to read, and his eyes fell directly on the phrase "Helping Hand."

When he had finished the letter and read the signatory, "DR. P. S. KISHORE," he put two and two together, recalling the young man who had phoned looking for a job. The touch of manners and character was exactly the type of intangible that can usher a candidate to the front of a queue. On Monday morning, January 17, Dr. Kishore had an interview. After that, he was the new two-week interim physician at Boston's Washingtonian Center for Addictions.

When the time had come and gone, Kishore had done so well and was so well liked that they created a new full-time position for the family physician on staff. He only grew more indispensable from there. Only a year later, when Dr. Lewis accepted a Chair at Brown University, Kishore had already proven himself as a replacement for director. He would fill this role for the next two years.

The Washingtonian Center and Dr. Lewis's work both influenced Kishore in a unique way. The Washingtonians had been a temperance effort in the 19th century helping alcoholics through direct engagement in small sobriety groups and individual accountability. The groups grew very popular but waned and fragmented into various competing interests. Their movement disappeared by the late 1800s, but not before it left a few addiction recovery institutions bearing its name in major cities, including the one in Boston. By the time Kishore arrived on the scene, the mission of addiction care remained, as well as an ethic that was not afraid to think outside the box in the interest of advancing patient care. In this regard, Kishore's new home provided him with a wonderful private research library in its basement with records and resources on addiction care from the early 1800s to the latest scientific research.

Dr. Lewis himself had contributed to this ethic and the resources. Beginning during his first residency in the early 1960s, he teamed with a famous psychiatrist, Norman Zinberg, to study heroin addiction. Zinberg's research and studies of heroin usage among Vietnam veterans would lead to the understanding that heroin addiction was not merely a physical problem, but social. Soldiers had, it was theorized, adopted heroin only to compensate while in the bleak, alienated condition in Vietnam. Of those who became addicted, almost 9 out of 10 shook it and readjusted to normal life, heroin-free, once reestablished socially back home.

In addition, Dr. Lewis also disapproved of treating drug addiction like a crime, but promoted addressing it as a public health concern. He would later advocate to end the War on Drugs and replace it with treatment through an "addiction maintenance" model of care.

Without ever planning it or perhaps even giving it a thought, Kishore found himself a natural home at the Washingtonian Center. His background was in family practice, which focuses on patients' families and social units, not isolated individuals. This naturally fit with the Washingtonian tradition of sobriety as a social accountability issue. It would also track naturally with the work advanced by Lewis. Treating addictions as a health and social concern more than an individual criminal matter dovetailed nicely, and formed a foundation for viewing addiction treatment through caring for and treating the whole person, physical, mental, psychological, spiritual, and social—not just the physical.

Kishore extended his outlook to his staff. Addiction medicine as a specialization or field was virtually unknown at the time, with only a couple of researchers like Lewis engaging it. Little attention was given to it, with most doctors heading toward more exciting and promising fields, and addiction treatment left to the fringes. In this state of affairs, there was very little in the way of professional development or continuing education for it, either. Kishore simply produced his own for in-house use. He would spend research time in that basement library not only advancing his own understanding, but writing a newsletter through which he would train and update his nurses and staff in the same advances. Little did he realize he was laying the foundations to pioneer in a field and have a broader reach in the community.

Kishore quickly gained valuable experience, and in a short time was being asked to help where there was need. Early during his career at the Washingtonian, Kishore was asked to give supplemental training on addiction treatment to physicians at Massachusetts Correctional Institution in Bridgewater, an old and massive complex of correctional institutions in Massachusetts, with separate facilities treating general population prisoners, sexual offenders, mental health inmates, and more. Addictions were on the rise among the inmate population, and help was needed. Kishore was more than adequate to address the problem.

The relationship developed at Bridgewater could not have been more fortuitous for Kishore, because the future of the Washingtonian was soon in jeopardy. The following year, a growing effort to centralize healthcare in the state inched its way forward. Smaller, privately-funded healthcare centers were disadvantaged as state-funded healthcare options grew. Despite the fact that more diversified options may often have provided more specialized, effective, and higher-quality care, they would be pushed out by the ever growing influence and power of the State "Department of Health and Hospitals," in conjunction with growing infusions of federal and state funds.

Over time, as private options struggled against their behemoth competitor, they would be absorbed into larger state hospitals under the auspices of helping them remain solvent. The Washingtonian Center was swallowed in such a scheme, which would later culminate in 1988, when governor Dukakis announced the first statewide "universal healthcare" plan. Centralization, however, always has other consequences. The ever-burgeoning and intrusive State Department leaguered the Center with regulations, inspections, and codes which forced costly changes. For an operation that for over a century, historically ran on the thinnest of shoestring budgets, and in order to help some of the poorest of the community, it did not make any sense.

One report noted, "Almost from the day the hospital was founded in 1857 by the Washingtonian Society of Boston, it achieved a reputation of being high on caring and low on funds. But with the era of charity care long since passed, the hospital was still providing $300,000 in free care annually. Last December [1979] it became apparent that $250,000 was needed just to make payroll and pay back bills through early March."[1]

Those back bills had accrued in part because the State's demands caused the diversion of a significant percentage of vital operating cost. A previous report revealed that the financial problems resulted when it took steps to "improve its safety measures" which were "made necessary to meet licensing requirements" imposed by the State of Massachusetts. It explained that "the hospital was forced to spend money it had hoped to use to expand the facility to attract more patients and more aid."[2]

The Boston Globe added this specter: "There is no other hospital in the state providing services comparable in patient cost to those at the Washingtonian. No one knows where the 1200 to 1500 inpatients who were annually admitted to the facility will go in the future."[3] To this number could be added that many more outpatients who would be left with no aid from the state hospital system at all. This sad tale would be retold later in Kishore's story.

The Boston Globe covered the work of the Washingtonian and Dr. Lewis during these years, taking an interest in the rare model

1. Jean Dietz, "Where Will They Go? Hospital for Addicts Closes," *The Boston Globe*, March 23, 1980, 45.

2. Peter Mancusi, "Oldest addiction hospital planning to close Friday," *The Boston Globe*, March 2, 1980, 31.

3. Jean Dietz, "Where Will They Go? Hospital for Addicts Closes," *The Boston Globe*, March 23, 1980, 45.

which provided detoxification care and interest in the patients' social environment, which the Center saw as vital to recovery. Providing substitute "maintenance" drugs such as methodone were important, but if given alone risked creating one more costly addiction.

Those who could not afford care could end up in worse scenarios. As the Washingtonian faced imminent closure in March, 1980, the *Globe* reported,

> "It's been cut off before," said one man, who drives 40 miles to Boston to drink his daily dose in cherry-colored syrup. "When I get it, I work. When I'm on street stuff, I have to hustle. Nothing violent. I specialize in silent house jobs when I need money."[4]

Dr. Lewis's early collaborator, Dr. Zinberg, also maintained a column in the *Globe*. Later the following June, when the closure of the Washingtonian had begun to be felt by those it affected most, a reader wrote in to ask why drug addiction treatment had left patients hanging. Their own brother was addicted and they feared he would end up on street drugs with the programs no longer available. Zinberg wrote back, lamenting the end of more informed and effective treatment programs for something that did not seem to serve the interests of patients themselves. He concluded, "What is happening is somehow political, for it has no medical validity."[5]

Crime rates and suicide rates among the addicted would only increase after the state system eliminated specialized care, especially among the poor.

The Washingtonian was therefore absorbed and eliminated by the system, and its model of treatment was left to atrophy and disappear. The business was soon bankrupted, but through a recent agreement, its building and property had to be forfeited. It was

---

4. Jean Dietz, "Where Will They Go? Hospital for Addicts Closes," *The Boston Globe*, March 23, 1980, 45.

5. Norman Zinberg, "Addict suddenly feels abandoned," *The Boston Globe*, June 8, 1980, 136.

sold off, and its former patients all absorbed into a much less effective, but highly profitable, model through the large hospital.

Kishore's training lectures to the prison doctors, then, established a relationship that would open yet another very needed
door for him.

Three

Beginnings of a Revolution

Around the same time Kishore joined the Washingtonian, he entered Harvard University to study for a master's degree in Public Health. He developed relationships with several doctors and professors working in the same area and with a similar philosophy of addiction treatment. Dr. Lewis had already inculcated a lifelong interest in addiction medicine. Likewise, at the Washingtonian, director Cleo Lachapelle had mentored Kishore further in Hospital and Healthcare Management. At Harvard, Kishore also encountered the concept of Global Public Health under Nobel Laureate Thomas H. Weller, recognized for his work in tropical medicine. Andrew Spielman, a specialist in Malaria, taught him about Public Health campaigns. Lecturer John Wyon encouraged humanitarianism in medical practice, and encouraged Kishore in the practice of community diagnosis. Here also Kishore studied under department head David D. Rutstein, a leading advocate of preventive medicine, and met Dr. Hugh Fulmer, who advanced the concept of community-oriented primary care. Finally, he learned sociological aspects of addiction as well as innovative research methodologies from Dr. William McAuliffe.

Concepts and ideas such as "preventive medicine" and "community oriented primary care," developed in this environment, would

15

echo later in Kishore's own work and his public advocacy as well. When he would eventually establish a private practice, he would in fact name it "Preventive Medicine Associates."

Kishore was already transferring some of these ideas in his lectures at Bridgewater, and his influence and direction bore fruit both for the institution and him. The fit was so natural that when the Washingtonian was submerged, Kishore found a safe and productive home at Bridgewater. For the next 13 years, he would flourish as the Associate Medical Director of the whole Massachusetts correctional system.

In 1979, Bridgewater had also contracted with Goldberg Medical Associates for staffing the necessary positions. Kishore met the owner, family physician Ronald Goldberg. Doctor Goldberg was skilled and successful at the business of Healthcare, and the resulting lifelong friendship further augmented Kishore's skillset in yet another area. Goldberg taught Kishore some finer points of contracts: writing, negotiating, upholding, and enforcing. The magnificent operation that would later grow under Kishore's model and leadership owed much to Goldberg imparting to him the art of enterprise.

Many of these skills Kishore developed and implemented to improve the medical care program at the facilities and help it to flourish. Working with Goldberg, he regularly staffed 60 to 70 part-time doctors to serve between 1400 and 2000 person-hours per week, 24/7, caring for hundreds of inmates in all branches of the system: mental health, sexual deviance, and general prison.

He also transferred the care he had shown in developing staff at the Washingtonian Center. Prisons can understandably suffer from high turnover rates in medical help, especially when the prison work is a side job for many of the doctors. The first signs of difficulty, liability with difficult inmates, etc., and most doctors who have enough challenges in their primary career already would not want to deal with it. Under Kishore, however, they stayed on. Kishore led them in broader areas of training: trauma care, advanced life support, psychology.

In addition, he took the lead in difficulties, acting as a buffer of liability for the doctors. For example, very common issues with inmates were asthma and seizures. As a result, some prisoners may complain about complications with being moved, requiring certain beds, taking certain medicines, etc., because of their unique constraints. Doctors did not want the additional liability thrust upon them. Kishore positioned the healthcare administration of the prison to assume responsibility for the decisions made by the doctors. Doctors felt protected, so more of them stayed. Where the attrition rate for prison doctors may average eight to ten percent normally, Kishore helped bring Bridgewater's down near one percent.

Two events coincided in the late 1980s, however, that would disrupt Kishore's practice again. In 1987, Massachusetts governor Michael Dukakis ran for U.S. President. Dukakis had supported very liberal rules for criminals, allowing even the most violent to receive educations and other leniencies like weekend furloughs. In the course of his national campaign, a major scandal erupted when the case of convicted murderer William Horton hit the media. Horton was serving a life sentence, but while out on one of Massachusetts's weekend furlough programs, left the state and was arrested and convicted of kidnapping, assault, robbery, and rape. He remains in prison in Maryland today. The news caused a major upheaval in the press, may have cost Dukakis the Presidential election, but also drove a major reaction in the state as well. The successor-to-be, Bill Weld, turned tough on crime preceding the 1990 election. His campaign rhetoric soared. He said he would "reintroduce Massachusetts prisoners to the joys of busting rocks," and be "to the right of Attila the Hun on crime."[1]

Once in office, however, not much changed in practice aside from minor tweaks in the laws. Furloughs continued. What changed drastically, however, was that the new administration moved to

---

1. Quoted in Jeff Jacoby, "Will the real Bill Weld please stand up?" *The Boston Globe, April 12, 1994*; www.jeffjacoby.com/874/will-the-real-bill-weld-please-stand-up

save budget cost at the expense of those who had the least public voice and reputation, those who could do the least about it: the prisoners. They cut the prison budget by 25 percent.

In the same years, Dr. Goldberg had suffered from a heart condition. He could no longer keep the operation solvent under such drastic cuts, and had far less capacity for the political battles. He and Kishore could no longer operate the system safely.

In succeeding years, the state awarded prison healthcare contracts to large national corporations that would provide streamlined, assembly-line type services at lower costs. The community primary care model was ushered out on a wave of politics and money, a note that unfortunately seems to become a refrain.

Kishore stayed to help transition the facility to the new workers, doing what he could to ensure the same standard of care until he left. But he had to look to the future. He continued working with Goldberg for a time, but also began to lay the foundations of a private practice. The contacts and relationships he had developed, and the reputation he had established in addiction treatment, would soon pay dividends.

***

Methadone treatment for addiction had been introduced under President Nixon as a stop-gap measure. The rise in drug use in the 60s and 70s created the great scare nationally which the President in 1971 called "public enemy number one." Soldiers returning from Vietnam were addicted to heroin in high rates. The whole nation was on alarm. Methadone treatment had been further developed in the early 60s, and by the time the alarm hit, methadone seemed like the obvious and most promising alternative. Addicted individuals would be diagnosed and prescribed medically-supervised doses of methadone. The new drug was safer than heroine, and a few patients even gained enough control to kick the habit altogether, eventually not needing the methadone either. Others would relapse. Still others, however, would continue on the new drug indefinitely, but at least they were in a safer environment. It was still controversial. Advocates argued that it saved lives, lowered crimes rates, and reduced transmission of infectious diseases (still the official argument today). Critics argued that it replaced one addiction with another, only at taxpayer expense, that methadone itself was dangerous, that there were other alternatives. As much remained to be learned and developed about addiction treatment at this time, however, methadone seemed to be a quick fix for Nixon and his War on Drugs.

The seminal efforts of men like David Lewis and Norman Zinberg, and later Kishore and others, on addiction eventually began to gain some traction. These men had blazed the trail, laboring in fringes of medicine; but in 1986, the American Medical Association had recognized the need and was calling for the creation of a specialty in addiction medicine.

Hospitals soon arrived at the same juncture on the demand front. More and more people were seeking medical help for addiction, but the avenues of treatment had all been centralized into the large hospitals. This meant that the medical establishment needed adequate answers. Again, Methadone was the standard, and it was mass produced, waiting for prescriptions in assembly line fashion. The late 80s and early 90s were seeing a tremendous number of cases flooding hospitals.

This came with inquiries of how to pay, and that triggered Medicaid and Health insurance industry discussions as well. As early as 1981, the Reagan administration loosened federal regulation on federal aid for substance abuse and mental health treatment. The change meant that states would get "no strings attached" block grants of federal money.[2] In 1992, the Massachusetts health care finance bureaucracy added a regulation for addiction care, almost certainly as a liability issue. The agency required any hospital with addiction treatment program to maintain an addiction care specialist on staff, at least in order to get coverage.

---

2. See Richard A. Rettig and Adam Yarmolinsky, eds., *Federal Regulation of Methadone Treatment* (Washington, D.C.: National Academy Press, 1995), 164 note 10; www.nap.edu/read/4899/chapter/8#p200064678960164001.

The AMA, however, had only put out the call for a specialty a few years earlier; there were not many doctors yet who could fill the role. In Massachusetts, Kishore was among the very few. As a result of the new regulation, he received call after call. Out of 73 hospitals in the state of Massachusetts, Kishore eventually ended up on staff in 30 of them, including some of the most prominent, such as Brigham and Women's, and Beth Israel in Boston.

The development allowed Kishore to maintain contacts and build a further reputation as more and more people could learn that his own developing model of care exceeded the state methadone assembly line model in quality and results.

The centralized powers developed as well, however. A regional group started in 1984 in New York City, and by 1989 it put on a national face as the American Methadone Treatment Association (AMTA). Throughout the 90s, this grew into a powerful political lobby. By 1991, a number of states had chapters, and by 1993, AMTA was publishing "State Methadone Treatment Guidelines." By setting "guidelines" for every state, the lobby effectively centralized control of drug advocacy for addictions, and mainstreamed methadone treatment. From a bird's eye view, the organization looks like a front for big pharma to sell its drugs to mass markets through streamlined, Medicaid-funded channels. This optic was enhanced when new drugs were developed, such as Buprenorphine (Suboxone®), and the organization changed its name to cover those as well: the American Association for the Treatment of Opioid Dependence.[3]

Fast forward a few decades, and the continued centralization of government powers over health care with flowing streams of billions of dollars will only create trouble of all kinds. If the love of money is the root of all evil, one can only imagine the evils that would befall. The confluence of massive, unprecedented government funding with corporate power, bureaucratic regulations, and powerful lobbies will result in making prescription-writing a top priority. For patients, this means personalized treatment will face

---

3. www.aatod.org/about-us/organizational-history/

intense pressure from a streamlined, one-size-fits-all assembly line approach: line them up and prescribe them methadone. Next!

***

After leaving Bridgewater, Kishore accepted positions with the various hospitals, but also continued applying and developing his treatment methods in private practices. This occurred in two venues. He founded Preventive Medical Associates (PMA) in 1991, but it would take a couple of years before getting fully credentialed and building the business. On a second front, Dr. Goldberg, post-illness, continued business as well, only scaled back somewhat. Kishore helped him in the meantime and gained valuable experiences that he would apply to his model.

The two had already begun as early as 1989 working through a private practice called Home Free, providing private, home detox services. Unlike virtually anything else Kishore had done, this service had a wealthier clientele. Fees could run $3,000–4,000 for home visits and one year of after-care, but clients were more than willing to pay in order to recover from addiction and yet keep the whole process private and confidential, at home, thereby avoiding unnecessary disruptions with jobs, contacts, friends and others who did not know and the client may not want knowing. Kishore was involved in around 200 such cases over a few years, and the experience taught him valuable lessons.

The first lesson came from the unique aspect of entering the homes of the addicted. The social aspect of an individual's addiction had long been a reality for Kishore even from his days at the Washingtonian. It was all the more real here. In dealing with an addicted individual, you must simultaneously address those in relationships with them. This includes attention to how the individual affects those around him or her, but also how the spouse, children, friends, etc. may also be affecting the addicted as well. Perhaps there are multiple addictions in the house. Perhaps there is enabling or codependency. There is always more than one person involved, and this must be taken into account.

The second lesson was observing the difference made from empowering the individual to address the cues and triggers in their own environment. These could include food, stress, schedules, and more. When a person is taught to recognize and identify, they can also be taught to cope. Empowerment here helps patients become self-efficient, and leads them to realize they must regain mastery of their own destiny. Instances of success make markers to compare to the past and realize progress. Overcoming the triggers that cause relapse means the guilt of relapse will be gone as well.

Thirdly, a vital aspect to sobriety is restoring relationships of love, and doing so is strongly aided when the medical party can take away from a spouse or loved one as many burdens, stresses, etc. regarding the medical aspects, and allow the spouse to focus on traditional expressions of relationships: serving, loving, normal life, etc. It helps reestablish the addicted person in a new paradigm of normality.

Kishore worked in the home detox model until 1996, but he would soon find reason to adapt it further. The majority of his home detox patients were from wealthier areas outlying the city. In the Greater Boston Area, the majority of patients could not afford this treatment. He had to adapt his model from home detox to outpatient detox. He would have to take the family values aspects of what he had learned and was practicing, and apply it to an outpatient setting.

In order to meet this challenge, Kishore did work directly with family members during treatment as much as possible. He also developed a system and a network of what he called SSPs ("special support person"), individuals who help keep the patient accountable and help them where needed. They help them make appointments, give them rides, reminders, etc. If he could not bring the practice into the family's home, Kishore could bring the family into the office, or substitute a family. These humble servants on his staff, or volunteers, were a key to the success of his system.

And succeed it did. This model of care increased exponentially in popularity and effectiveness. "Gangbusters" would be putting it lightly. In just a couple of years, PMA expanded into two full floors of office space. It was positioned as a leading provider in the state; so much so that in 2001, Blue Cross awarded PMA their statewide contract for addiction care in Massachusetts. With a total of 2.4 million members under coverage, the Blue Cross contract translated to thousands of potential addicted patients per year. Kishore grew his staff and facilities to meet the need. Other contracts followed.

Kishore's approach helped the insurance company as well. While an initial outpatient addiction visit could normally run $400 or more in a psychiatric setting, in primary care it would cost much less. Further, Kishore's clients wrote letters to Blue Cross themselves to praise his effective and affordable practice. Things added up quickly for the insurance company.

For Kishore, it was never about the money. He in fact paid himself only very modestly. After many years of developing his career, it was clear he had a calling and a mission. He began to get even more serious in implementing it. He aggressively entered the highways and byways, seeking out the addicted. He knew he had a better answer than methadone-type treatments. He knew he could save many who were being overlooked or even exploited. He developed relationships with safe houses, sober houses, church ministries to the addicted and the homeless, and much more.

Over the next decade, Kishore would grow from a single office to a network of 52 clinics throughout the state, treating hundreds of thousands of clients. At this point, it seemed like the sky was the limit. Little did Kishore realize, he was quietly making some powerful enemies. In the meantime, however, Kishore was revolutionizing addiction care. Most people cannot imagine how sorely this was needed.

Four

A New Level of Care

After decades of learning and practice, Kishore created and developed a revolution in addiction care with proven results in long-term sobriety. His model appears in stark contrast to a mediocre, but well-financed, status quo in which some benefits are claimed, but the patient remains on a substitute narcotic, possibly for life, and more negative aspects of the reality are swept under the rug.

The tragic but unavoidable dose of reality about mainstream addiction treatment in America comes in the following facts: there are no standards of success, low standards are accepted as "evidence" for "effectiveness," and even with what meager standards are in place, talk of success in treatment is largely avoided, probably because the overall reality is so depressing. *Sobriety* is not even discussed. The best that is usually imagined is that a patient hopes to regain some functionality in life while remaining on opioid replacement drugs indefinitely. Kishore raised the standard from the status quo of "methadone maintenance" (meaning, stay on this replacement drug indefinitely) to "sobriety maintenance" (meaning, get sober and stay that way).

In the few cases where we can compare his results to those available from mainstream treatments, Kishore's model flips matters nearly on their head. Under traditional models, around 80 percent of addicted patients relapse in the first month, and only about 6 percent remain on the addictive treatments long-term. Under his personal, intensive model, however, Kishore was able to achieve sobriety rates around 50 to 60 percent after one year on average.

"Sobriety" is the key word which makes the contrast in statistics all the more staggering. One would think that when considering the *treatment* of addiction, the end-goal would be *sobriety*. Would common sense not dictate that when treating addiction, we should measure ultimate success in terms of the rate of long-term sobriety of the patients or clients? Granted, we could discuss stages or steps along the way, but the end goal *should* be for the treatment to render the patient drug-free. This was certainly Kishore's goal, and he achieved it at a rate unseen anywhere else in the history of addiction treatment.

This is nowhere truer than when viewed in comparison to the prevailing models of medication-assisted treatment (MAT), with methadone, buprenorphine, or similar addictive opioid replacements. In these models, *sobriety is not even discussed.* If maintaining a patient on state-controlled replacement drugs instead of street heroin or other opioids results in lower crime rates, and other beneficial effects for the limited number who remain in treatment, then that is usually considered the best possible result, and accepted indefinitely. This is the outcome for which major drug companies lobby, provide medical experts, and push legislation for well-funded government programs. Yet you will rarely if ever hear discussion of sobriety.

This is true not only regarding the opioid crisis, but substance use and addiction in general. Some addiction treatment programs that do consider sobriety do not consider the crucial first month in their sobriety statistics. In a research survey created for internal use only, Alcoholics Anonymous, for example, skipped the first month completely. Yet the majority of its recidivism rate is accrued in that window. Beginning at day 30, their average sobriety rate for five surveys over a twelve-year period (1977–1989) was only

19 percent. This means that of those who began the program, 81 percent had quit within *the first month*. After a year, 95 percent were gone.[1]

Other addiction treatment and rehab centers acknowledge this problem. Some claim high success rates, but only after redacting heavily and counting only select cases in their own favor. Failures are blamed on the patients or other factors. Other centers may claim more modest recovery rates like 30 percent. Even these, however, only count those who actually finish the program.

This problem was recognized in a *Washington Post* article on August 8, 2010:

> Controlled studies of specific treatment centers are rare; compounding the problem, many programs simply don't follow up with former patients. And when they do report a success rate, be it 30 percent or 100, a closer look almost always reveals problems. That 100 percent rate turns out to apply only to those who "successfully completed" the program. Well, no kidding. The 30 percent rate applies to patients' sobriety immediately after treatment, not months or years later. . . .

> A recent review by the Cochrane Library, a healthcare research group, of studies on alcohol treatment conducted between 1966 and 2005 states its results plainly: "No experimental studies unequivocally demonstrated the effectiveness of AA or TSF [12-step facilitation] approaches for reducing alcohol dependence or problems." . . .

> In a 1990 summary of five membership surveys from 1977 through 1989, AA reported that 81 percent of alcoholics who began attending meetings stopped within one month. At any one time, only 5 percent of those still attending had been doing so for a year. . . .

---

1. See figure C–1 from "Commentary on the Triennial Surveys (from 1977 to 1989)," AA internal document 5M/12-90/TC.

The Washington Post article ended on an interesting note, similar in tone to Kishore's basic approach: "In the end, there is simply no need to remove alcoholics from the support of relatives and friends and shut them away for the customary month in rehab."[2]

When we consider how these statistics are fudged, we return to the grim dose of reality. Something like a whopping 80 percent drop out along the way, especially in the first month, and they are excluded from the stats. The claimed 30 percent recovery figure then really represents only about 6 percent in actuality. This is consistent with what figures we can glean regarding opioid treatments as well, except they remain on the replacement.

One of the few studies that gives a long-term picture of the reality is an actual natural history of heroin addicts published in May 2001. After following the lives of 581 heroin addicts for 33 years, the study showed virtually no sobriety that could be attributed to any treatment program. At the last tally, a meager six percent were in methadone maintenance. Meanwhile, around 22 percent had achieved abstinence spontaneously or through self-seeking. Two percent reported occasional narcotic use, 7 percent reported daily use, 4 percent were in jail, the whereabouts of 12 percent were unknown, and 48 percent were deceased (some of these were through age, but many were related to drug or alcohol use or implicated health concerns).[3] A 2005 essay by the same primary author, with others, noted that while "Nearly all studies" affirm the effectiveness of methadone treatment, "the beneficial effect of any single treatment episode is often short-lived, and relapse to drug use is common." It also noted that most studies also ignore alternative treatments and how they can succeed.[4] A yet more recent journal article noted the need to account for the social dimensions

---

2. Bankole A. Johnson, "We're addicted to rehab. It doesn't even work," *The Washington Post*, August 8, 2010.

3. Hser Y, Hoffman V, Grella CE, Anglin MD. A 33-Year Follow-up of Narcotics Addicts. *Arch Gen Psychiatry* 2001; 58(5):503–508.

4. Yih-Ing Hser, Douglas Longshore, Mary-Lynn Brecht and M. Douglas Anglin, "Studying the Natural History of Drug Use," in *Epidemiology of Drug Abuse*, ed. by Zili Sloboda (New York: Springer, 2005), 36.

of an addicted individual's life, and developing long-term strategies of chronic care, reaching across social and health care systems, to intervene in the patients' experiences.[5]

These are all tacit, or in some cases explicit, acknowledgements that the opioid replacement treatment models are a failure, or a first baby step at best. They are all also advances Kishore had incorporated into actual practice decades ago, and had been practicing when the state shut him down. It is not surprising to find that such academic advances cite earlier work by Kishore's early mentor, David Lewis (and others). Lewis's work in 2000 in a major medical publication asserted and defended the view that addiction is not merely an individual health care problem, but a social problem, and must be addressed long-term in the whole social live of the addicted.[6]

Where academia showed signs of slowly coming around (with the help of a select few nudges), Kishore was blazing trails in actual practice and having stellar success. The social scope of the patient's life, the multidisciplinary thinking, the detailed, holistic interventions, the long-term strategy—Kishore had honed and refined all of these and more through extensive experience with thousands of cases.

How He Did It

Kishore accomplished what he did by doing what any scientist of any stripe ought to do: observe the problems, ask scientific questions, and look for scientific answers. He focused his attention on the 900 pound gorilla in the room. It was what some other models quietly accepted as collateral damage, the cost of doing business, or at best what they quietly swept under the rug. Kishore pulled back the rug: what about those 80 percent who drop out in the first month?

5. Hser YI, Hamilton A, Niv N., "Understanding Drug Use Over the Life Course: Past, Present, and Future," *J Drug Issues* 2009; 31(1):231–236.

6. McLellan AT, Lewis DC, O'Brien CP, Kleber HD, "Drug Dependence, a Chronic Medical Illness: Implications for Treatment, Insurance, and Outcomes Evaluation," *JAMA* 2000; 284(13):1689–1695.

Why are the vast majority dropping out? Is it really inevitable? Can something be done to prevent it?

For Kishore, it was not about making one drug or program look good versus others; it was about serving people and saving lives. So, he focused on that massive neglected group. His observations would pay off.

Over time, Kishore realized that the first four weeks of treatment followed very predictable patterns with recurring traits. Moreover, these patterns and the issues that arose within them were treatable or preventable with simple family-practice and community health solutions.

He broke down the four weeks and their unique challenges week-by-week. (While more detailed versions of this process can be found elsewhere,[7] this brief report is enough to show the rare combination of practicality, grit, character, and genius found in Dr. Kishore.) During the first week after detox, the addicted patient experiences post-acute withdrawal syndrome, which has many symptoms, some very intense. Instead of merely replacing the addiction with methadone or similar narcotic prescriptions, Kishore drew from his background in family practice and treated symptoms such as nausea, vomiting, diarrhea, restless leg syndrome, profuse sweating, mood swings, and more all with non-narcotic prescriptions.

When beset with severe cravings, he provided injections of naltrexone (Vivitrol®), which is a non-narcotic opioid blocker. This means it decreases the cravings for opioids. Originally approved for alcoholism, it also showed promise for drug addiction as well, it had just not yet been approved directly for that. A primary care physician, like Kishore, however, could prescribe it for use, a perfectly normal and legal thing doctors can do; and he did, effectively.

Kishore, in fact, was a pioneer who helped the later approval of naltrexone for drug addiction as well. Before the FDA approved it for this use in 2010, Kishore had already been using it off label for drug addiction for at least four years. His analysis of the case series compiled between 2006 and 2010 were posted at the

---

7. From compilation provided Martin Selbrede, Chalcedon Foundation.

American Association of Treatment of Opioid Dependence (AA-TOD) Conference in Chicago. During this time, Kishore actually asked to be audited to provide financial and professional regulatory accountability; but the fringe benefit of the intense oversight was that it helped to verify his sobriety rates of nearly 60 percent.

Today, the National Institute on Drug Abuse (NIDA, a branch of the National Institute of Health) publishes on its website a research report that affirms, "A NIDA study showed that once treatment is initiated, a buprenorphine/naloxone combination and an extended release naltrexone [that is, Vivitrol®] formulation are similarly effective in treating opioid use disorder." The difference is that unlike methadone or buprenorphine (brand name Suboxone®), the Vivitrol® is non-narcotic and non-addictive. In other words, while gingerly walking a line that could inflame powerful pharmaceutical lobbies, the federal government nevertheless acknowledges that non-addictive naltrexone is at least as good. Today, even the Wikipedia page notes it has benefits over its narcotic competitors.[8]

Such a major contribution seems like a capstone to one's career. For Kishore, such achievements became not only routine, even like stepping stones to the next one, but he also remained grounded enough to realize the major limitations of any single element. Naltrexone was a crucial advance, but it was only a minor one in the big picture. Addiction treatment includes *many* other factors than even a core prescription. Many of these would be social, and many would start to kick in within the second week.

During this next week, the individual's own mind wages war upon him or her. They may have overcome initial withdrawal symptoms. Now they begin to rationalize that they can control their old habit. They may try small amounts again. If left alone, such mind-processes can lead to relapse. Here is where Kishore acknowledged the vital need for *community*: group support from sponsors, professionals, or recovered addicts, becomes crucial to

---

8. As most recently accessed (September 18, 2019): "It has benefits over methadone and buprenorphine in that it is not a restricted medication." en.wikipedia.org/wiki/Naltrexone

countering the power of self-deception regarding control. Kishore learned from much older, previous models on this point, but he went above and beyond. He staffed many such sponsors, professionals, and volunteers who could provide 24/7 support if needed. A strong support network would remain crucial into the third week. After about two weeks had passed, the patient's old social network comes calling. This could include former dealers, friends who are also users, other environmental triggers—many things. Misery needs company; active addicts can grow jealous of a freed one. If the patient had themselves been involved in dealing, they could now become the subject of revenge. Dealers have various tactics of persuasion. They use gift bags of "freebies"—free doses to lure the patient back into the "enterprise." If the carrot fails, they have the stick. They threaten violence: personal harm, or worse, to rape one's mother or sister. They may even offer a "hot shot"—a freebie laced to kill.

It is precisely here, when temptations with friends or offers of free drugs are thrown repeatedly in the individual's face, that Kishore has the naltrexone ready. This helps tremendously to break the power of what those old relationships have to offer. Meanwhile, the support network, as well as faithful friends and family, work to replace the old community, and replace the environment in which the addiction could flourish.

The support network remains vital into the fourth week, when the most devastating killer attacks the patient's spirit: loneliness. That old environment brought with it the drugs, but also a sense of familiarity, comfort, and even security and identity. It was a circle of friends, so-called, and a sense of who one is. Stripped from this, and in a whirlwind of change, the patient can feel alienated, isolated, and alone. At such a point, they loose self-esteem. They may contemplate suicide. The patient needs the sense of meaning and purpose, and identity, provided by a new, sober community.

Kishore supplied these needs not only through his unique support networks, but also by preparing the individual potentially to become part of it. He works with employers and family to maintain the patient on a regular schedule. Others could be plugged into community service, vocational training, or be trained as ambassadors or sponsors in Kishore's network itself (depending on the case), all the time using "trust but verify" principles of ensuring unbroken sober state through detection technologies with either urine, saliva, sweat, blood, or hair.

It was this few-weeks-long dedicated effort on the part of multiple parties, all under Kishore's experienced direction, that translated a patient from a bad condition in a bad environment to a much-improved condition in a safe environment.

Compare this to medication maintenance treatments which may have some benefits for some symptoms, and may even be paired with counseling or other activities, but in no time at all the individual is thrust right back into the same circle of friends, users, dealers, triggers, and everything else. They are right out of the methadone clinic and right back in the same circle of "friends" that got them in trouble to begin with—and they will have very little of a support group to fall back upon for help. This is why most never make it past the first month.

Kishore specifically targeted the problem of the 80 percent relapse rate during the first thirty days of addiction treatment. And he nailed it. He nailed it by realizing that addiction is not merely an individual medical problem, it is a *social* problem. Properly treating it, therefore, means much more than prescribing a slightly less addictive drug by which to cope. It means entering the whole life of the patient, treating their whole experience, changing their environment, providing them a new life, meaning, and identity. All of this requires a new community. Kishore supplied all of these, and he did so at costs far lower than other treatments available.

A Model of Models

Over the course of his vast experience, Kishore consistently drew from his own experiences as well as a variety of other models and efforts available. We have already mentioned his experience with various Harvard Medical School professors and doctors. We also mentioned his early access and use of the unique library at the Washingtonian Center for Addictions. His efforts, however, reached even further.

When the Washingtonian met its unfortunate end, Kishore was able to save a portion of its valuable library. He used it to found the National Library of Addictions in 1993, and eventually provided a permanent home for it in 2006 in Brookline, Massachusetts. By then it had grown into multiple floors, along with research offices, conference facilities, visiting scholar apartments, a community lab, and a prevention institute. It eventually expanded into three buildings. And it became much more than a traditional library.

Kishore also founded centers for studying Neuroscience, Addiction, Correctional Medicine, Addiction Law, Recovery activities, and Pharmacology. He partnered with the Massachusetts College of Pharmacy and American Board of Addiction Medicine to provide training programs through the college and the library. He also was in the process of creating a training program for pastors in collaboration with Rt. Rev. Samuel Hogan, an Instructor at Harvard Divinity School and Bishop of the Church of God in Christ.

Even more than this, however, the National Library for Addictions became both a community center for the practice and its patients, as well as a library with feet. Through its various resources and activities, patients and their friends and families and support groups strengthened each other. Those who became ambassadors and sponsors for the clinics would regularly go out from the library "headquarters" equipped like evangelists, taking literature and lectures to doctors and others in need of it.

In compiling knowledge and literature from all places, and not limiting himself to a narrow medical "orthodoxy" (no matter how powerful or profitable it could prove to be), Kishore was able to draw from various models, implementing their successes and adjusting for their shortcomings.

The first such model is known as the Minnesota Model. It appealed to Kishore in that it is a sobriety-centric model, focused on leading the addicted to a drug-free life. It had been designed in 1950, based specifically on Alcoholics Anonymous, to which it added a new blend of professional and trained non-professional care. It also included family involvement. The elements of community and sobriety appealed to Kishore, though he felt the model needed improvements. For example, it cleaved the addicted from their families and often does not allow the assistance of medications in maintaining sobriety.

In the 1990s, a rival approach emerged that replaced the twelve-step model with evidence-based medicine, specifically a combination of medication assistance and psychotherapy. It also recognized the complex nature of addiction, involving both personal and social factors. The early advocates of this system used naltrexone, though methadone was not ruled out. It sought also to replace the rigidity of the Minnesota Model.

Kishore realized that he could draw good elements from both of these models without pitting the two as utter one-or-the-other rivals. He combined the focus on sobriety and support groups in the first, and the allowance for naltrexone and medications in the other, as well as the recognition of social factors in both.

Even from the similar methadone "maintenance" model, Kishore drew a nugget of inspiration. The concept of maintenance is not wrong in and of itself, even if we recognize that merely replacing one addiction with another is not the answer. What it gets right is the need for maintaining the patient in a course of improvement over a period of time. It is the *goal* that needs improvement here. So, Kishore changed the idea from methadone maintenance to *sobriety* maintenance. Let's help the patients get actually sober, and then maintain them in that lifestyle until they are free on their own.

This goal, of course, means a long-term involvement in the patients' lives and development. To this end, a third model helped as well. A Florida-based model applied clinical help while patients lived in apartment-style housing and maintained daily tasks and jobs. This was closely related to the "Clubhouse Model" pioneered in New York, and with which Kishore had been familiar through an example in Worcester, Massachusetts. These models keep patients on close medical care and supervision, as needed, while providing a sense of home, normality, real life. It humanizes the person and allows them to maintain work and get involved in various activities, schooling, vocational skills, employment support, and more. It creates a therapeutic community; it makes community itself a method. "I love that model!" Kishore exclaimed in a private interview.

Kishore integrated all of these good features into his primary care model. To these, he added advances and innovations to make his clinical care even more effective, and individual primary care for every step along the way. As he would once put it, "To be a good addictionologist you need to have 18 to 20 disciplines under your belt. You must be a good primary care doctor, you must be good with behavioral sciences, you must know toxicology, clinical pharmacology, psychology, you have to know social sciences and you have to know the law."[9]

Innovations for Better Care

Kishore not only revolutionized the first four weeks of treatment, his model applied to a full year of care and beyond. In the second month, he helped patients begin to clean up the wreckage of the past and plan for their future. This included personal mentorships, in-person meetings, to set new boundaries, higher standards, and higher expectations for their lives. In month three, the body returns to something more like normal, which can actually bring unsettling realities, especially for women. These simple but important physiological changes are met by remedies from simple primary care.

Likewise, the process of recognizing cue and triggers for addictive behaviors continues. Kishore's practice matched these needs with equally intense attention, prepared to bring support. It is almost like babysitting in a way, but is still a crucial service to get the patient more into the clear.

Kishore explains how this intense personal attention is both key and virtually unique in the addiction treatment world. "My

9. "Q and A with P.S. Kishore, M.D.," *M.D. News, Greater Boston Edition,* September 28, 2007.

peers don't want to invest this much time in an addict's life, but the reality is that an addict is surrounded by things that will pull them down. Nobody recognizes this. You have to be there with them to know this, and to treat them accordingly."[10] The addiction treatment must be social and *present*. It must be *there*, walking through the valley of the shadow of death with the addicted. This must continue, Kishore says after much experience, for at least a year if not five years observed by a physician. Sobriety is a life-long process.

The need to be present with the weakened or broken individual, with a goal of actually getting out of *this* valley, drove Kishore to innovate and develop ever more powerful aspects and nuances to addiction treatment. One fundamental aspect of traditional treatment is urine testing. The reason is simple. Heroin leaves metabolized morphine in a user's system for up to three days. Periodic testing can reveal if an individual in treatment has "relapsed." But Kishore noted key shortcomings with the conventional system, so he moved to fix them. He moved from a "deterrence" model, which virtually punishes patients, to a more specific "detection" approach, which helps the patient and focuses on treatment.

First, traditional urine testing is designed to catch only what it categorizes as "relapse." It assumes from the three-day window that testing need only be done at a maximum of twice a week. If it lasts for three days, there is no need to incur the extra effort and expense of testing every day or two. Makes sense. But this assumption misses a couple things as we will see in a moment.

Second, the conventional model sets a fairly high threshold for the amount of drug that must be detected before it is considered a relapse. This may derive from the general purpose of methadone maintenance: to help people cope enough to live their lives, and especially to get back to work. The state and its preferred model do not want to be in the business of striking out every single patient with strict standards and rigorous testing schedules, thereby pulling loads more people out of the workforce. It is better to limp

10. Quoted in Selbrede, 15.

along than upset the flow of things. This also has the consequence that patients are not getting branded as failures immediately, or regularly, and at best being required to start all over.

Kishore, however, looked deeper than a one-size-fits-all standard. He also observed that if an individual's drug use is caught early enough, it could be treated as a temporary slip instead of the dreaded full relapse. Further, such cases could be caught by more frequent testing, and with methods designed to detect trace amounts or to discern more refined measures of the targeted substances. Employing his trademark individualistic approach to each patient and their environment, Kishore was eventually able to determine which patients in which settings required closer supervision. In some cases, more frequent testing was required; in others with better supervision, less frequent testing than the conventional models was needed.

In order to implement these findings, Kishore developed his own quantified testing standards and opened his own testing labs to handle the hundreds of thousands of patients he would see. It was an in-house operation designed to serve Kishore's clinics in the most accurate and efficient way possible. He could not rely on outside labs to provide either the degree of testing or the precise timeframes his methods required.

Ironically, when all averaged out, Kishore only prescribed testing around 2.2 times per patient per week, which is right at the conventional standard. However, because he determined that some patients need three to four times per week (though others may only get one or none) the state focused here when it first tried to find ways to charge him with wrongdoing (no evidence was ever produced on these grounds, and no charge was ever brought; the state later switched to charges of a kickback scheme and billing fraud, neither of which were ever proven either). It seems unimaginable that a minor innovation in urine testing which had hardly any noticeable increase in frequency of testing on average would become the fulcrum by which a government would shut down the largest and most successful addiction treatment in history.

Conclusion

We have barely scratched the surface of the revolution in addiction care which Kishore effected. The long personal development in various areas of medicine, addiction care, correctional care, public health, healthcare management, healthcare *business*, private care, primary care, insurance companies, regulatory issues, psychology, social factors of patients' lives, the dangerous aspects of the drug trade, and so much more, all of which had to go into the equation of Kishore's life and achievements, would probably take multiple books to relate. But as Kishore himself says, "Ideas do not come *de novo*." It takes much experience and in places, poking around as if a blind man with a stick, making small increments and steps here and there. There are many such steps and details we have had to leave out.

What we see, however, is a man fully devoted to his care for others, and further consumed by the need always to improve his care and service. Often times, this included decisions that came with great personal cost. Kishore could easily have toed the party lines, kept quiet, practiced the status quo, and made much more money than he ever did. But he thought outside the box.

Thinking outside the box in this case led to success rates that conventional addiction treatment could only dream about. Even more, it led to a *standard* of what success is that medication-assisted treatments do not even consider, for it is not even on their radar. On all fronts, Kishore's advances in treatment beat both tradition sobriety models and conventional medication-assisted models. Most sobriety models, when they are not moving the goal posts, have to admit they lose 80 percent of their patients in the first month. Methadone assistance models do not even talk about *sobriety*.

Kishore provided a non-addictive alternative to the latter, and elevated the sobriety treatment to the tremendous rates we have seen. There has never been anything else like this. It is a revolution in addiction treatment and care.

Five

Triumph and Trial

The revolution in treatment and care came with tremendous success, but it came also with a tremendous personal cost. It almost seems like a Cain and Abel story. The one did what is right and realized success. The other's failure turned to deadly envy when they looked at the successful in their midst. Fear and rivalry grew into murder in his heart. The brother came to be seen as a rival, an enemy, that must be crushed. Kishore was probably naïve that his success and his advocacy for success could be stoking such malicious ambitions among rivals that could include powerful governments and corporations.

In the meantime, Kishore's success only grew. As the addiction epidemic spread, so did demand throughout the state. To meet the demand as it arose in various population centers, Kishore used ZIP code analysis to place new offices in the most strategic places for efficient service. By 2007, he had expanded in 17 locations. Only three years later, that number was 27. Eventually, he would reach a height of 52 clinics or branches in every corner and population center of Massachusetts.

These offices not only provided the most efficient access points for growing demand, they also functioned to expand the reach of Kishore's community and provide a network of care for his long-term patients. On one occasion, for example, a man who had newly reached sobriety took a vacation on the Cape, hours from Kishore. The man stepped on a foreign object at the beach and was in terrible pain; but he feared to go to the Emergency Room for fear that they would prescribe him narcotic painkillers that were popular and notoriously addictive. He called Kishore who simply informed him not to worry, he had a clinic literally down the road from his vacation spot. He could administer primary care for the foot, and prescribe something fitting for his patient's condition as recovering from addiction.

Kishore's effectiveness and growing popularity fed each other and gained national attention. He was recognized and awarded for his many contributions by virtually everyone that gives relevant awards, except mainstream establishment parties, who saw him as a growing rival. For example, on November 21, 2004, the Boston Celtics honored him with their "Heroes Among Us" award, which they give to acknowledge "individuals who have made an overwhelming impact on our community, positively affecting the lives of others."[1] Among other things, the website to this day acknowledges his work and the tremendous reach of it: "Dr. Kishore is often referred to as the 'Doctor of Addiction Treatment' for his efforts in the development of treatment methodologies. He has worked with over 140,000 drug addicts throughout the past 15 years."[2] Kishore was even recognized, along with other recipients of this award, by his Senator, the late Ted Kennedy, in the Congressional Record.[3]

In May of 2010, Kishore was elected as a Fellow of the American Society of Addiction Medicine. This honor is reserved only for those whom the Society decides "have made major contributions to the quality of American medicine."[4] Only a year or so later,

---

1. www.nba.com/celtics/community/heroes_2004_11.html
2. www.nba.com/celtics/community/heroes_2004_11.html
3. Sen. Ted Kennedy, "'Heroes Among Us' Award Recipients," *Congressional Record—Senate* (2005), S6726.
4. "West Roxbury's Dr. Kishore honored by American Society of Addiction Medicine," May 2, 2010; roslindale.wickedlocal.com/x57972235/West-Roxburys-Dr-Kishore-honored-by-American-Society-of-Addiction-Medicine

the State would be breaking in and arresting this same fellow. The list of honors goes on. Between 1994 and 2001, Kishore received awards from hospitals, the Massachusetts Medical Society, community groups, churches, Healthcare support groups, conservative groups (Newt Gingrich's American Solutions for Winning the Future), area promotional groups (Boston Event Guide's "Thirty Extraordinary Bostonians"), a pharmaceutical company, as well as The Association for Multidisciplinary Education and Research in Substance use and Addiction.

Perhaps even more ironically, in the thick of the era in which some state officials were formulating how best to take Kishore down, within months of the SWAT-storming of his house, the federal government in the form of the Centers for Disease Control was seeking out his expertise. On March 22, 2011, he answered the call to address a CDC conference. He presented a paper on "Epidemiology and Surveillance of a Disease State in a Primary Care Practice" which discussed his experience in how "primary care practices can be at the forefront of local and community issues."[5]

Medical journals and publications grew interested in his success with addiction. An illustration in *M.D. News* in August of 2010 featured Dr. Kishore's practice and the uniqueness of his methods. Its conclusion impresses:

> Dr. Kishore's multidisciplinary approach to drug and alcohol detoxification and sobriety maintenance now reaches over 250,000 people in Massachusetts. They have close to 10,000 visits per month and Dr. Kishore plans to expand his reach into neighboring states in the future. Offices are open seven days a week and people are seen immediately without regard to insurance. After they are started on treatment, the office will work with them to get the coverage they need.

---

5. "Local Doctor Punyamurtula Kishore Presents at the Centers for Disease Control and Prevention (CDC) 28th Annual BRFSS Conference," March 31, 2011; www.pr.com/press-release/309993

When you meet Dr. Kishore and the people that work in his preventive medicine treatment centers, you can't help but be impressed by their level of dedication, enthusiasm and compassion. His approach to treating drug and alcohol addiction is evidence based and scientific, but it also benefits from a healthy dose of common sense and hard work by people who care very much about what they are doing. That is a good combination for treating any illness.[6]

The numbers are mind-numbing in regard to the sheer size of the operation, as well as what they mean for patients in terms of the resulting sobriety rates. They are *ominous*, however, when you realize what diverting a full third of the potential patients in the state—hundreds of thousands—from the establishment addiction industry's line of cashflow. That is a huge blow to what otherwise could be called a well-oiled, easy-money machine.

None Dare Call it Corruption

Such a money machine has costs that exceed money. Recall that at this point, Kishore has an intimate view of the drug ecosystem (legal and illegal), the criminal justice system, public health systems, marketing and business systems, the state regulatory system, the health insurance industry, and more. While he had some darker aspects yet to learn through hard experience, he had experience enough to see how the assembly-line-like medication maintenance system fit into a larger interlocking series of industries. Collectively, as he put it, these systems interlock to make up a "Wheel of Death" from which few of the addicted escape without proper treatment.

More than just a trap for the addicted, the Wheel of Death includes a powerful web of special interests, political lobbies, and more, which work to protect their power more than any single thing. While illegal and prescriptions drugs proliferate and the

---

6. Christopher Iliades, "The Many Facets of Addiction," *M.D. News, West of Boston Edition*, August 28, 2010.

opioid and addiction epidemics run viral, the prevailing view is to treat addiction as a crime, or that it is a disease from which so few can recover that the least of possible evils is to keep them on a state-approved drug indefinitely. These approaches mean that we clog the courts and fill the prisons with drug offenders, while powerful drug companies lobby legislatures to cover their own addictive narcotics on state insurance plans. Then, the addiction treatments along with an army of desks with brass name plates wait like vultures for multi-million-dollar federal block grants to be handed down from Washington, D.C. When the chunk of cash arrives, various groups and industries are waiting to carve it up and devour as big a share as they can get. The mainstream media helps the system by highlighting the problems of epidemics and announcing the approved remedies, but rarely will you hear a peep about the nature of the system, where the millions and sometimes billions are flowing, the damages done, the poor success rates, the lack of sobriety and accountability, or the alternatives that are providing real success right in their own back yards.

Rarely if ever, for example, does mainstream media highlight the astounding fact that virtually every State currently spends more money on addiction and substance abuse than almost any other line item in their budgets. Education is usually the only exception. According to the New York-based nonprofit Center on Addiction, states spend on average around 16 percent of their entire state budgets on addiction and substance abuse. Massachusetts spends a whopping 22.2 percent.

Massachusetts this year passed a $43 billion budget. Twenty-two percent of that will equate to about $9.5 billion spent on preventing, treating, maintaining, and trying to clean up the wreckage of substance abuse and addiction. As far as the official line items go, the majority of this is spent on the latter aspect: the drug war, policing, corrections, health care, mental health, and welfare and child assistance for broken families and the unemployed.

Vague line item categories in budgets, however, are easily abused. This is especially true when bureaucrats, lobbies, and other special interests have spent years training themselves in ways to appropriate funds from one area for their own desires. Aside from the direct millions flowing to buy the actual replacement medications and to pay the clinics prescribing them, the Mental Health industry is right there in tandem. It was early on recognized that methadone or buprenorphine/Suboxone® replacements alone were not enough. But whereas Kishore employs an army of family, group, community supports and primary care 24/7, the regulatory powers-that-be determined that behavioral therapy (visiting a psychiatrist) would suffice. Then they lobby to get mental health care for the addicted covered by state insurance as well. Next thing, the millions start flowing to the psychiatrists, too. Then social workers worked their way in as well under the guise of "Behavioral Health."

The appropriations run rampant especially when the federal government, through its Substance Abuse and Mental Health Services Administration (SAMHSA) branch of Health and Human Services, hands down tremendous block grants to the states to fight addiction. The latest budget includes $1.9 billion in block grants for "prevention and treatment," another $1.5 billion for "State Opioid Response Grants." This latter category claims to spearhead a "five-prong strategy" to fight the addiction crisis. But the five prongs include these: "regulatory activities, ongoing training, certification, and technical assistance to provider groups and communities impacted by the opioid crisis." You can sum most of these under the *single* prong heading, "bureaucracy." In other words, billions go into the states for vaguely-defined purposes, and an swarm of bureaucrats, politicians, and special interests are standing there waiting to carve and devour the funds as they see fit.

You may think some of this money, logically, covers the actual methadone and buprenorphine treatments; but no. Those get their own direct grants: an additional $89 million specifically for that.

You may think perhaps it covers the mental health part of the machine. No, that gets its own line, too: $722.6 million worth, *plus* another $150 million just to expand and open *new* behavioral health clinics that do not yet exist, another $115 million yet specifically for children's mental health, *and* another $102 million for mental health education programs. There are also plenty of millions for other purposes beyond these.

Massive as it is, this is all still small beans. The federal government releases a "National Drug Control Budget." The number continues to balloon year to year, up from just under $14 billion in the first year of the Obama administration to $27.8 billion in 2018, and a whopping $34.6 billion projected for 2020. Grants from this money get distributed through Health and Human Services (HHS) as well as the Department of Justice, Homeland Security, Veterans Affairs, and the Departments of Agriculture, Defense, Education, Labor, State, Housing and Urban Development, and the Treasury. "It has tentacles in every place," Kishore said.

Taken together, the Center for Addiction's 2005 report noted substance abuse and addiction costs federal, state, and local governments a combined total of nearly half a *trillion* dollars.[7] These numbers are now a decade and a half old. Impact costs have certainly risen with inflation at least, as well as in proportion to the epidemic. The Massachusetts state budget has increased by about 80 percent since that time.

From the perspective of the average individual, such numbers represent a tragedy of hurt, pain, suffering, and crime. They are a warning sign that something needs to be done. To some people, however, the same numbers represent only a massive stream of revenue. They are huge, flashing, neon dollar signs. Here is an opportunity to raid the coffers, raid the kitty, by providing "goods and services" for government billions. Further, since the government is the key player, this means law, policy, and monopoly can force out competition from free market advances, improvements, innovative technologies, more effective private treatments or charities, and more. Moreover, it will have the power of authorities and much of the media at its disposal.

---

7. *Shoveling Up II: The Impact of Substance Abuse on Federal, State and Local Budgets* (New York: The National Center on Addiction and Substance Abuse at Columbia University, 2009).

Much of this narrative only discusses the more mainstream ways powerful lobbies and bureaucrats can work. Once all the various appropriations, especially block grants, get made, the creativity at state and local levels can really get started. For example, SAM-HSA announced in February 2019 that HHS would be collaborating with the U.S. Department of Agriculture to provide subsidized rural housing for the addicted in treatment.[8] Likewise, there are discussions occurring in which some advocates suggest addressing the substance abuse in homeless communities by using government funds to provide so-called "tiny homes."

Similarly, beginning in the late 80s, the federal government designated five major urban areas as "High Intensity Drug Traffic Areas," and provided some targeted funds to them. Within a decade, such designations had spread until it was easier to count places in the nation that were not so designated; and the funds spread likewise. Today, these "HIDTAs," as they are called, are further channels through which funds flow to state and local law enforcement, health, and mental health for substance abuse reasons.

Another outstanding example is the move in some states to appropriate funds to stock the opioid-blocking drug Narcan® (naloxone, not to be confused with naltrexone) in schools to treat potential overdoses. Ironically, the executive director of the National Association of School Nurses said the move was a "community decision," but that sounds odd coming from the head of a lobby that is pushing for the measure. The same article notes that the company that makes Narcan® previously gave the School Nurses' Association a $25,000 grant. It is also giving free samples to schools in collaboration with a program with the Clinton Foundation.[9]

On top of all of this, the Trump administration has declared the opioid epidemic a "Public Health Emergency" since the Fall of

---

8. www.samhsa.gov/newsroom/press-announcements/201902151000

9. Ken Alltucker, "Naloxone can reverse opioid overdoses, but does the drug belong in elementary schools?," *USA Today*, Sept. 11, 2018; www.usatoday.com/story/news/nation/2018/09/11/schools-fighting-opioid-epidemic-overdose-reversal-drug-naloxone-narcan/1210383002/

2017. According to an NPR article covering the move, this opens FEMA resources and further Medicaid funds for use in substance abuse issues, to fund methadone and buprenorphine medications and to waive regulations to make them easier to distribute, to re-direct federal personnel to the new emergency, and other channels of funds and resources.[10]

In Kishore's Massachusetts, the money machine in the addiction treatment industry grew obviously with the epidemic. A Boston. com article from 2011, when Kishore's practice was at its height, related that the state health department had spent $325 million treating addictions with methadone or Suboxone® (most with methadone). The article notes that the average cost per patient for methadone treatment was nearly $20,000 per annum. Consider-ing that the cost of the actual basic methadone by itself is only a few hundred dollars per year, one gets an idea of how much money gets consumed in the state health, mental health, and administra-tive and regulatory systems.[11]

Ironically, that long article was an advocacy piece promoting the superiority of Suboxone® to methadone. It took space to highlight alleged corruption and kickback schemes in 12-step programs and praised the state's attorney general for sniffing them out. Perhaps some of this musing was true for other cases. Nevertheless, when it comes to the treatments involved, even this article ended with a note of inadequacy:

> Like methadone, the long-term maintenance use of Suboxone doesn't address the underlying causes of addiction. But it does give addicts an opportunity to

---

10. Alison Kodjak, "What Could Happen if Trump Formally Declares Opioids A National Emergency," *NPR*, August 11, 2017; www.npr.org/sec-tions/health-shots/2017/08/11/542767898/president-trump-to-declare-national-opioid-emergency

11. Lawrence Harmon, "Under the influence of methadone," *The Bos-ton Globe*, Boston.com, May 15. 2011; archive.boston.com/bostonglobe/editorial_opinion/oped/articles/2011/05/15/under_the_influence_of_methadone/?page=3

succeed in behavioral or talk therapy. Suboxone won't
fill the "hole in the soul" of addicts, as identified by 12-
step programs, either.

The fact is, even the better of these drugs and their methods *do
not lead to sobriety very often at all*. In fact, both drugs are abused,
and both keep the addicted on a new addiction for years.

Those who favor Suboxone® have no problem pointing out this
evil with methadone, especially when administered in private, for-
profit methadone clinics. The previous article cited one case in
which a woman spent 25 years on methadone treatments:

> She, like many addicts, describes her years on metha-
> done as an endless cycle of daily dosing and metha-
> done-related appointments. Tucker, who received
> state-subsidized treatment, said she sought to reduce
> her dosage, but staffers told her not to concentrate on
> the milligram number, just on how she felt.

> "The for-profits keep you so high, you don't know
> what you're doing," said Tucker.

The case is hardly out of the ordinary, but the common experience that comes with it is even more discouraging:

> The worst part, she said, was the daily experience of
> being around other addicts who weren't committed to
> recovery. "This is the best place to hook up if you want
> to do dope," she said.[12]

Suboxone, however, faces similar problems. Already in 2011, the
Portland Daily Sun reported the experience state drug officials and
police were encountering:

> Katz cited Suboxone as the latest drug to be abused.

> The trend is particularly unnerving because of Sub-

---

12. Lawrence Harmon, "Under the influence of methadone."

oxone's importance in treating opiate addiction when used for its intended purpose. . . .

Potential for abuse with this drug has been completely underestimated and has exploded, she said. "There seems to be an unstoppable flow on the street."

Why the underestimation? A huge part of the blame lies in letting the foxes guard the hen house. Officials believed the promotional material the drug manufacturers themselves told them:

"Pharmaceutical companies assured everyone it couldn't be abused. All the information came from pharmaceutical reps," Katz said.[13]

The cogs of the "Wheel of Death" are apparent nearly throughout.

Of Truth and Power

Kishore had long since understood the limitations of the prevailing piecemeal approach using medication and limited mental health care. It suffers from an odd case of tunnel vision and a "whack-a-mole" approach, as he puts it. So, while he sees methadone and buprenorphine as "good" drugs, they have a very limited place. Any treatment that truly desires to help patients and stem the epidemics of addictions will have to acknowledge these limitations or else keep failing at the increasingly deadly rates we are seeing.

For this reason, Kishore consistently advocated a more holistic, primary care *model* of actual treatment over against the methadone model of addiction care, and he has always been careful to diagnose what is limited about the latter. In a 2010 interview, he noted that it was a matter of emphasis on results: "Replacement therapy certainly has its place and can save the lives of some individuals, but for a large percent of the population, sobriety maintenance is possible, and treatment strategies must be available for those who

---

13. Margie Niblock, "Suboxone abuse rears its head," *The Portland Daily Sun*, May 17, 2011; issuu.com/dailysun/docs/pds5-17-11

would like to get back to a drug-free life."[14] This was similar to the position he had stated a few years earlier in the same publication:

> It is not so much that Methadone is good or bad. It's the system that has evolved around it. We need Methadone. It is a medicine. There are some people whose damage has been such that they need a maintenance medication. The process whereby people have to go every day to pick up the medicine is not humane. Without checks and balances, however, the system can degrade very easily. Only about 18 percent of the patient population on Methadone actually stays true to maintenance modality. Many use other illicit and prescription drugs along with Methadone. It is a good drug, but there has to be good case matching and case management.

It was this "good case management" that Kishore had so painstakingly developed over the years. He had shown that it could be carried out just as effectively without the addictive replacement. This last quotation appeared in 2007, just after Kishore had started his polysubstance applications of naltrexone/Vivitrol®. By 2010, his model would be even more potent.

He also, however, did not mind openly criticizing that broader system in which methadone could be used in an assembly line fashion and with no outlook to sobriety. A 2002 article in a local paper, the *Woburn Advocate*, quoted him referring to methadone as "Uncle Sam's legal dope." That does more than highlight the medical aspects of the drug or alleged treatment. Whether intentional or not, such a phrase also calls into question the politics of it, which also means the politics of the funding of it. Invoking that realm is playing with fire, though it may also be just the right thing to question. Publishing his views critical of the leading mainstream models, however, would lead to strong and eventually tragic backlash.

---

14. "Q & A with Punyamurtula S. Kishore, M.D., M.P.H.," *M.D. News*, November 28, 2010.

Kishore unwittingly had established himself as a major threat to the addiction treatment industry. He had worked, trained, studied, and developed his practice all with some of the most renowned doctors, psychiatrists, and scholars in his fields. Since his very introduction to addiction medicine, he had worked within the more holistic method following the tradition of the Washingtonians. He had developed this method through various stages, after tremendous study, application, and experience; and he had done so with tremendous success.

As his success as a private clinician climbed rapidly, Kishore became more and more visible as an advocate—one could even say *activist*—for the method he developed. This meant taking an open stance against what he saw as a deficient treatment based in replacing heroin with other powerful drugs. This advocacy would draw unwelcomed, and powerful, attention.

In 1999, for example, Dr. Kishore posted an editorial in *The Boston Globe*, entering a public discussion about a potential methadone clinic in Nantucket at the time. He noted briefly that the "so-called methadone-maintenance approach" was not only expensive, but "it does not address the chronic nature of addition and ultimately does not adequately serve the public good." He was right. Those treatments do not seem to "address" the chronic nature of addiction so much as *exploit* it. Instead, Kishore urged, clinics should "consider a 'sobriety maintenance' program that stresses nontoxic substances, teaches coping skills, and tailors treatment to individuals."[15]

A response letter snapped back on behalf of the drug-maintenance treatment. It missed the larger point and objected as if Kishore were merely attacking maintenance treatment absolutely. It was an oddly narrow, yet strident, protest. Despite its defensiveness and a bit of tunnel-vision, the brief, scolding retort was undersigned by prominent directors of substance abuse centers in the Boston area.[16] It seemed like axe-grinding rather than calm,

---

15. Punyamurtula S. Kishore, "Nantucket's problem," *The Boston Globe*, October 10, 1999, p. 359.

16. Alan A. Wartenberg, Janice Kaufman, and Richard Slein, "Methadone

objective consideration, but it had big powers behind it.

This type of confrontation would escalate much further in an exchange that took place in 2006, as well as in its fallout, when Kishore published an unassuming and moderate response with the Partnership for Drug Free America. In March of that year, Kishore published an article in *The Boston Herald* titled, "Suboxone Catches On in New England." Suboxone was the new methodone. It was performing the same role and being prescribed similarly. Kishore made the same criticism as before: we must not rely on drug "maintenance" alone, but recognize it as one narrow aspect of a process, and that there is a method much better and more successful: primary care sobriety maintenance.

Doctor Jeffery Baxter of UMass Medical School answered in support of Suboxone® and medication maintenance treatment. He said that the addicted need drug maintenance like diabetics need insulin. He called Kishore's comments "complete ignorance" and "pure nonsense," yet he never interacted with the actual position, Kishore's practice, or a single word about his track record of success. It was clearly a hit piece.[17]

In his very moderate response, Kishore noted once again that maintenance medications do have a role, but the need is for something much greater, more intensive, and focusing on the individual's whole life:

> The few studies that have been done regarding the natural history of opiate addiction suggest that the largest segment of the surviving population of this lethal disease do achieve sobriety (22%). A much smaller group requires long-term maintenance medication (6%). Whatever path is taken, addiction treatment requires long-term rehabilitation with extended periods

---

and addiction," *The Boston Globe*, December 5, 1999, 318.

17. Jeffrey Baxter, "It's Time For Physicians To Support The Maintenance Model," jointogether.org, March 10, 2006; republished by the National Alliance of Advocates for Buprenorphine Treatment; www.naabt.org/newsletter/apr2006/default.htm

of outpatient treatment. In most cases in treating addictions, medications serve only an adjunctive role to the long periods of rehabilitation necessary. . . .

The maintenance model is an excellent harm reduction strategy. . . . This model, however, can potentially sell the addict terribly short, if it is invoked before the option of sobriety maintenance is fully explored. A treating physician must always have his or her patients' best interests in mind.[18]

The narrative from the other side clearly was already set. Kishore got a visit from a agent of the federal government's Substance Abuse and Mental Health Services. It became clear enough that interests behind the replacement drug sales were not happy with Kishore's views and that he should not speak out publicly this way again. That bureaucrat went on to become a manager with the big pharma company that makes Suboxone®.

Damming the Flow of Funds

One need only take a step back and look at the larger picture to see why these sides really clashed in the ways that they did. A further factor, perhaps even the primary factor, aggravating the powers that be was that Kishore's success meant they lost hundreds of thousands of billable patients to the evil forces of sobriety.

The most damaging thing to the addiction treatment industry is to have a competent individual get ahead of them with a competent system and simply inform patients to try a system of sobriety first. Some of Kishore's brochures simply beat the whole system by doing just that. One pamphlet outlined different "stages" in addiction treatment. Methadone and other maintenance medication treatments do not show up until stage two. Stage one was Kishore's primary care model, which led a majority of its patients to sobriety before the machine could even get a chance to get them hooked on

---

18. Punyamurtula S. Kishore, "Many Roads Lead To Recovery," jointogether.com, April 3, 2006.

a replacement drug. By the time most of them had gone through his stage one, they would never need stages two through five.

Through his amazing success with sobriety, however, and the dramatic growth of his business into hundreds of thousands of customers, Kishore diverted a large stream of revenue from the mainstream models, and in more than one way. The maintenance clinics and doctors lost business; the drug companies lost sales; the hospitals lost clients; and the mental health professionals were losing out.

Given the enormous percentage of government funds quietly flowing into the mental health industry for addiction purposes, it is no surprise that a complaint was lodged with Blue Cross on related grounds. Around 2007, during the six years Kishore serviced the Blue Cross contract for addiction treatment, the complaint came through that he was not referring enough individuals for mental health treatment. Ironically enough, Blue Cross actually pulled the contract. The result was not only that the insurance company would have to dole out more money to satisfy the mental health providers, but the poorly-organized transition ended up with much of the new referrals landing out of network. This cost them even more.

Meanwhile, Kishore is simply trying to help people actually get sober and drug free. He was not only succeeding, but he was doing so at tremendous discounts. In a 2007 article, the reality was recognized by a third party, an expert in health care accounting. *M.D. News* related,

> Pharrel S. Wener, Chief Operating Officer of Medical Business Management Limited of Boston, states that addiction treatment has become a huge industry. "What Dr. Kishore has done is to bring quality care to John Q. Public," said Mr. Wener. "Two thousand-eight-hundred dollars for a year's worth of care, compared with roughly $10,000 for a three-day inpatient detox makes a compelling case that patients, physicians and insurance companies can all relate to."[19]

---

19. "The Business of Addiction," a sidebar in "Q and A with P.S. Kishore,

The comparison here is only to in-patient detox. The numbers are far more astronomical than just that. Out-patient treatments make up the vast majority of cases, and while these may appear to come at more efficient figures, they do not. They come at a vastly greater volume to begin with, and we have already seen the tiny fraction of the cost that actually goes to unbranded cost of the drug alone. Volumes of millions end up in the pockets of providers, corporations, bureaucrats, and more.

Kishore was able to provide an alternative system of care, without addictive replacements, that led to real sobriety at very high rates, at costs far below what the other treatments required. What could there possibly be in this to oppose? The clear offense on his part was in preventing the flow of millions of dollars to those who were expecting it. For this, he was a threat that had to be eliminated.

M.D.," *M.D. News*, Greater Boston Edition, September 28, 2007.

Six

The Takedown

During the height of the success of his practice, trouble
would come literally knocking. Kishore answered a rare
knock on the door of his home at the peculiarly late
hour of 10:45 at night, September 20, 2011, only to be rushed
by a bewildering show of force. Armed SWAT members barged
through the door, guns out, shouting commands, taking over the
premises. They were there to serve search and arrest warrants at
the behest of the Massachusetts attorney general.

They had an overkill of force: helicopter, black vehicles everywhere, agents of all sorts, a K-9 unit. They ordered his wife to sit.
They made Kishore get dressed so they could haul him off. He
was marched to his room. While he dressed in front of them, one
demanded to know where he had hidden any guns, gold, or cash.
He had no idea what they were talking about. They led him to a
vehicle and roughly shoved him in, injuring his shoulder. It was a
rude beginning to an even rougher series of legal attacks to come.

Over the following four years, Kishore would be subjected to an
onslaught from state officials, lawyers, and the courts.[1] The state

---

1. A more detailed account of the insane charges, tactics, and trials that
followed over the next few grueling years is being compiled and provided by
others. Here, we only include the essential highlights.

piled up scores of counts of charges against him, but as he resisted with facts, rigorous documentation, and consistent legal remedy, the state was forced to drop the bluff charges; but they were not done. Intense pressure, stalling tactics, media smear campaigns, piles of legal costs, and even dirty tricks took turns, wave after wave, wearing down the senior doctor, slowly eroding his ability to mount any legal resistance. When his finances were finally exhausted and he could no longer pay attorneys, he was led as a lamb to the slaughter, alone, before the prosecutors and court yet one more time, literally in bonds, weakened and without hope, resigned to sign a guilty plea as the least of possible evils.

By this time, however, gone were the grand threats of life in prison. The plea deal included 360 days in county jail, probation, a restitution amount they know a broke man will never be able to pay, but most importantly, the main goal they were after all along: he was required to resign his medical license. This means the state officials and powers that be will not have to worry about Kishore damming up the flow of funds anymore. It means no more competition from successful sobriety. It means they burst the dam: the stream of addicted patients will no longer be diverted into primary care and sobriety, and the stream of government millions will flow once again into their own system.

It was not as if Kishore was a stranger to pressure, but he was naïve about the extent to which they would eventually go.

One of the first maneuvers was a subversive attempt in May, 2009, to resign his license for him though a lawyer on his behalf. The guy called Kishore out of the blue to announce this move, but Kishore rejected it. A few months later, a sober house invited Kishore to a business discussion. The proposal was not all that savory and after some time in discussion, Kishore backed out. Little did he know that the whole thing had been a sting attempt by the government. They were trying to nail him with bribery or kick-back schemes or some other shady dealing by partnering with a disbarred lawyer and a known subpar safe house. They failed, and this apparently angered the state more. Instead of recognizing an innocent man with higher moral standards than they themselves had, they pushed harder.

Next, they tried indicting Kishore via a grand jury, on charges of fraud, bribery and kickback schemes. Kishore had structured his entire business according to the authoritative National Association of Community Health Centers guides, and he kept lawyers on staff specifically to make sure he remained compliant. The state was on a witch hunt. The grand jury was just the place to get what they wanted. Defense arguments are not presented in grand juries. Prosecutors present a case to empaneled citizens for the purpose of getting an indictment. It is usually a one-sided affair with the state prosecutors having tremendous influence to get what they want. As one judge once said, they could get a grand jury to indict a ham sandwich if they wanted to.

Once the indictments were received as desired and the charges came, then it was game-on at the court level. Or so the state thought. It filed the most outlandish set of complaints in court, attempting to paint Kishore and his entire operation as utter quacks, a complete scam artist in it for nothing but loads of money. The filed complaint dismissed his long track record by calling him a "purported" expert. It completely dismissed his entire practice as "a façade of good works" which "masks a business empire wholly and single-mindedly devoted to maximizing revenues for Dr. Kishore and Defendants [the business]."[2] It went on to label the business a "largely unlawful enterprise." Perhaps most shockingly, it insulted Kishore by saying he exhibits "an utter disregard for patient welfare." No single person in Massachusetts had shown a greater regard for the welfare of the addicted than Kishore had for over 30 years—probably ever!

These types of exaggerated claims only serve to mask the weakness of the state's case. Further claims betrayed something of the grand narrative already discussed. They accused him of "strong-arming clients" into taking Vivitrol® injections because, they alleged,

---

2. *U.S. and Massachusetts v. Preventative Medicine Assoc.*, filed in U.S. District Court for the District of Massachusetts, 2–12–2010, p. 2–3.

he would receive "handsome compensation" from state health insurance and "incentives" from the drug's manufacturer. There was, however, never any compensation received. Unlike some physicians, Kishore did not stock and sell the drug himself. He had it ordered through the pharmacy and shipped directly to the patient. There was no chance for markups or compensation on his part. Further, Kishore believed it unethical to make profits in such ways. As multiple audits revealed, Kishore's largest expense was his payroll for around 370 employees, and his own salary was always well within the accepted range for a family practitioner in Massachusetts. Given that he was a considerably higher profile doctor with a medium-sized business of 370 employees, limiting oneself to an average salary speaks to his own sobriety, self-control, and humility. It also exposes the state's litany against him as utterly ridiculous.

As this first round of charges fizzled and the case fell apart, the state then used one of the legal tricks in its arsenal of plea bargain tactics. Plea bargains are routine, of course, but they are also routinely abused. Prosecutors can pile excessive charges just to intimidate a defendant, or they can tantalize the defendant with a lesser charge in exchange for something they want, information for example. Kishore's case is even more dubious. The state can offer a sentence that includes "self-monitoring" during a probationary period, an apparently lenient sentence. Such monitoring, however, requires a state-approved agent to monitor, usually the defendant's attorney. Given that this state-approved position is well-paid, however, it is in the defending attorney's self-interest to push his client to accept such a deal. This can effectively amount to the state buying off the defendant's attorney, compromising the attorney's loyalty to his client! Massachusetts attempted this pressure on Kishore's attorney in exchange for a guilty plea, but Kishore would not agree to it. That was January 2011. Only a few months later, another state official suggested a deal in which Kishore simply give up his testing labs and he could stay in practice. But his quantitative testing innovation was a central element of his success.

Then the blitzes came in rapid succession. In September, Kishore's public persona began to disappear from the internet: a Wikipedia page outlining his achievements disappeared. Kishore's 2006 *Boston Herald* article that sparked the ire of the pharmaceutical reps and the state attorney general was not only scrubbed from the internet, it does not even appear in the *Boston Herald* search archives. Then the SWAT raid came, and Kishore landed in jail. The next day, the state attorney general Martha Coakley held a press conference highlighting recent busts in Medicaid fraud, but she carelessly conflated facts. She accused his practice of stealing $20 million from the state of Massachusetts—a claim that was never substantiated, and for which the state never provided a shred of evidence.

Kishore was briefly released, but rearrested on the state's assertion that he may flee the country. They also sweepingly seized thousands of emails to comb for evidence, despite the fact that hundreds of them were between Kishore and his legal team—a violation of attorney-client privilege and the fourth, fifth, and sixth amendments of the U.S. Constitution. When Kishore's attorneys filed a complaint about this infraction, the state assured the court it was not reading the privileged emails it was not supposed to. The matter, however, was never resolved.

The case dragged on for the next three years, with continued pressure and relentless tactics from the state. They tried to have his license revoked through the state Board of Registration in Medicine. They dragged and postponed court dates. They interrogated multiple former employees trying to dig up dirt. They initiated fresh investigations for the same purpose.

The cases were always weak and even the dirty tactics could not prevail, but the trials nevertheless bankrupted Kishore. His personal finances were exhausted, and the business was emptied, his properties liquidated. Even the National Library of Addictions, that fabulous research and community center, did not escape. Thousands of patients were left without care and the state was sent scrambling trying to find treatment for them.

When Kishore's resources were drained, his attorneys abandoned him. He was exhausted. He had watched his practice and career be destroyed. His situation looked hopeless. The state pressured him to sign a plea. It was only to one charge: one count of larceny over $250. The allegations of kickbacks, bribes, false claims to Medicaid, and others were never proven and never could be proven, and in fact Kishore's company no longer even existed. It took the destruction of the man's business by the full force of the state, and the destruction of his image in public through smear campaigns and misinformation. Once a guilty plea was finally extracted, it immediately hit the headlines. Even a British medical journal carried it, and nevertheless was still parroting the conflated claims about "complex kickback scheme" and "millions of dollars" that had been poured into the media early on.

Not surprisingly, the alleged kickbacks of which his company was accused stemmed from a practice that is widely known and used by other clinics and labs throughout the state. It is a preferred practice by authorities to rent space in the sober houses as part of a contract to perform testing for that house. There is nothing controversial about it—unless someone on a witch hunt wants to pretend there is in any given case. And when they do, apparently, no one is safe.

The claims about fraud were accompanied by media allegations of overly-frequent testing and overcharging. We have already discussed his innovation in testing, and that he nevertheless averaged the same as everyone else. As for overcharging, the prosecutors claimed he would charge $100 or $200 per test, but this case was never proven, and with the plea never had to be proven. It turns out, the opposite was the case: Kishore came in below the market standard for the cost of testing.

When the dust is settled, it is clear that an innocent man was railroaded by the bureaucracy, and who knows what other special interests were involved? But this tragedy is worse: this is not your average innocent man. This man had created a revolution in addiction care that changed the lives of hundreds of thousands of patients in a way no one else does. When you look at Kishore's life and career, the things that most stand out are not greed and avarice, as the state recklessly portrayed. They are instead his own selfless addiction to caring for people and improving how he can care for people.

His fault lies not in kickback schemes or frauds, but in tirelessly outperforming his competitors. His energetic work in securing contracts with sober houses was not a scheme to cash in, but a feverish attempt to save patients before they fall into other systems that would have them hooked on methadone or something similar for years instead of heading toward sobriety. Kishore worked to reach those people first, and it appears the state considered this type of "theft" unforgiveable. It had to be stopped.

For that "crime," Kishore was attacked, beaten down, and lost almost everything. Today he is impoverished, a convict, and bereft of his medical license. The state of Massachusetts destroyed the most successful addiction treatment anyone has even seen, and precisely at a time when the opioid crisis seems to be not only growing, but spiraling out of control.

Yet for all of that, Kishore is down, but he is not out. His focus is not so much on the evil others have done to him, but on what good he is still able to do for those suffering from addiction. There is more to come.

Conclusion

Looking Forward

You would think that Kishore is now left a broken man, without hope, with nothing left to do but sadly nurse his wounds and live out a meager existence. You would be wrong. Through all of this, he has not even bent slightly toward morbid introspection or self-pity. His focus remains on those in need, the addicted, his mission—and he remains optimistic.

Kishore is looking to the horizon, planning and developing what he can do next. He is still an academic with a background in public health. He has 40-plus years of experience leading the addicted to sobriety. He still travels often and lectures out of his extensive and unique knowledge of treating addiction. His is already rebuilding an educational network of Health Centers in Maine. He still impacts the lives of many people who need help, and those who are helping others as well.

Is it possible he could rebuild what he had done before? Can he practice medicine elsewhere? Can he set up an international center? Addiction is now a growing epidemic also in the state of Punjab in his native India. According to Kishore himself, education about addiction and its treatment must become a priority. "We must educate ourselves first," he says—"ourselves" being physicians and public health leaders. "Otherwise there is no leadership. There are no generals in the field." The lean into military terms highlights once again that the problem is not only the addiction itself. He adds, "There is no one to fight against the cartels of addiction care." Given the chance, Kishore can certainly develop the proper educational programs for doctors, but will that be enough, and will he even get that much of a chance?

Only time will tell. Yet another possibility, however, is that Kishore may yet ultimately be fully exonerated. He has kept records throughout his case. With the changes in Washington, there is a rumbling about desires to undo what many see as the damage done in the wake of Obama-era upheavals like the Affordable Care Act. It is certainly possible that a sudden, self-serving crackdown on a rival health care system in the nation's most socialized state health care system immediately after the passage of ObamaCare was not entirely a coincidence. With greater centralization of power coming down the line with more money and state-run "marketplaces" established, it could very well have been an added imperative to move against impediments like Kishore's model.

Whether anything will come of any rumblings among the Trump administration or not, the need for Kishore's knowledge and influence can certainly not be denied. Some kind of comeback is needed whether with a helping hand from the federal government, or whether Kishore is able to rise from the ashes in a more local, organic, holistic fashion.

Kishore's story right now does not end with justice. In that sense, it does not yet have a happy ending. History, however, moves forward. If justice comes, Kishore will certainly enjoy it. If it does not, he is already actively creating a new place where he can help, and moving forward there, anyway. He is actively attending and presenting at conferences and informing other physicians and community leaders. Moreover, a growing support group of diverse talents is forming around his views. He is optimistic, and he will not stop fighting to fulfill his mission.

Punyamurtula Subbarao Kishore, M.D., M.P.H.

Notable Achievements and Accolades

1. National Merit Scholar, Republic of India, and State Special Scholar, State of Andhra Pradesh – 1967

2. Appointed Acting Medical Director of the Washingtonian Center for Addictions – the oldest continuously operating Addiction Program in the United States – 1978

3. Appointed Associate Medical Director of the Commonwealth of Massachusetts, Department of Correction Facilities – 1980

4. First in the country to initiate a "Home Detoxification Program" for Substance Abuse – 1989

5. First in the country to establish a comprehensive National Library of Addictions comprising 14,000 volumes of books – 1993

6. First in the country to provide "Sobriety Maintenance" program for the Addicted Community – 1996

7. First contracted statewide Medical Consultant for Blue Cross Blue Shield/Magellan, the largest insurer in the State of Massachusetts – 2001

8. Recognized by the Boston Celtics as a "Hero Among Us" for contributions to the treatment of the addicted – 2004

9. First to establish a comprehensive "Neuroscience Center" to delve into the neuro psychiatric and pharmacological complexities of Addiction Diagnosis and treatment – 2008

10. First in the country to develop a comprehensive new "Model of Care" for the addicted, presented as the "Massachusetts Model of Addiction Treatment" at the National

Institute of Drug Abuse Blending Conference in Albuquerque New Mexica – 2010

11. First in the country to use Injectable Naltrexone (Vivitrol®) successfully to reduce cravings and prolong the "Sobriety Maintenance" experience—successfully bringing it to the market place – 2010

12. First in the nation to establish a residency-training program in Addiction Medicine for physicians in a private practice – 2011

13. First in the country to provide comprehensive Primary Care-based lifelong Addiction Care over a large geographic area, to a large number of people, at a reasonable cost, over a long period of time—serving close to a quarter of a million members – 2011

14. First to establish church-based Health and Healing Centers to provide vetted information to faith-based communities – 2012

15. Elected Distinguished Fellow of the American Society of Addiction Medicine – 2015 (Previously elected Fellow 0f the American Society of Addiction Medicine – 2010)

16. First to establish "Community Education Centers" to provide health education to the populations in different states – 2016

17. Aided the Commonwealth of Massachusetts in all branches of government: Executive (Governor's Special Advisory Panel on Forensic Mental Health – 1989); Judiciary (Judicial Committee, Supreme Judicial Court Substance Abuse Project Task Force – 1995); Legislative (Testimony before Committee on Mental Health and Substance Abuse – 2011); and Administrative (Advisory Board Member, Mass Health Primary Care Clinician Plan – 2002–2011).

Contact Information

Joel McDurmon
Author
P.O. Box 371
Braselton, GA 30517
jmcdurmon@gmail.com

Punyamurtula S. Kishore, MD, MPH
"The Doctor of Addictions"
P.O. Box 67070
Chestnut Hill, MA 02467
860.936.7900
psk@pmai.net

Further Resources

Hero in America: Dr. Kishore and the Epidemic of Greed.
A documentary, directed by Joaquin Fernandez,
Forthcoming; www.heroinamerica.com

Made in the USA
San Bernardino, CA
10 July 2020